T0190162

Register Now for Online Access to Your Book!

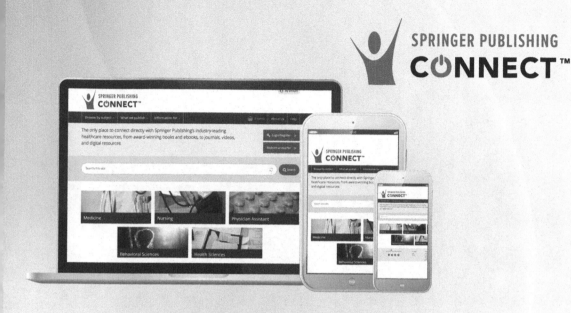

Your print purchase of *The Well-Managed Ambulatory Practice* **includes online access to the contents of your book**—increasing accessibility, portability, and searchability!

Access today at:
http://connect.springerpub.com/content/book/978-0-8261-5663-1
or scan the QR code at the right with your smartphone. Log in or register, then click "Redeem a voucher" and use the code below.

A5RKRFUD

Scan here for quick access.

Having trouble redeeming a voucher code?
Go to https://connect.springerpub.com/redeeming-voucher-code

If you are experiencing problems accessing the digital component of this product, please contact our customer service department at cs@springerpub.com

The online access with your print purchase is available at the publisher's discretion and may be removed at any time without notice.

Publisher's Note: New and used products purchased from third-party sellers are not guaranteed for quality, authenticity, or access to any included digital components.

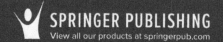
SPRINGER PUBLISHING
View all our products at springerpub.com

Register Now for Online Access to Your Book.

CONNECT

Scan here for quick access

THE WELL-MANAGED
AMBULATORY PRACTICE

Elizabeth W. Woodcock, DrPH, MBA, FACMPE, CPC, is the founder and principal of Atlanta-based Woodcock & Associates. She has focused on ambulatory practice management for more than 25 years. She has led educational sessions for a multitude of national professional associations and specialty societies and consulted for clients as diverse as a solo orthopaedic surgeon in rural Georgia to the Mayo Clinic. She is author or coauthor of 17 best-selling practice management books, including *Mastering Patient Flow* and *The Physician Billing Process: Avoiding Potholes in the Road to Getting Paid.*

In addition to her consulting work, she serves as an adjunct assistant professor in health policy and management at the Rollins School of Public Health of Emory University. In 2011, she founded the Patient Access Collaborative, an invitation-only coalition of 90 academic health systems and children's hospitals dedicated to patient access improvements in the ambulatory enterprise. She has served as the executive director since the organization's initiation.

Dr. Woodcock is a fellow in the American College of Medical Practice Executives and a Certified Professional Coder. In addition to a Bachelor of Arts from Duke University, she completed a Master of Business Administration in healthcare management from the Wharton School of Business of the University of Pennsylvania. She earned her Doctorate in Public Health (DrPH) from Johns Hopkins Bloomberg School of Public Health.

Mark J. Bittle, DrPH, MBA, FACHE, is a senior scientist in health policy and management at the Johns Hopkins Bloomberg School of Public Health. An experienced healthcare executive, Dr. Bittle is board certified in healthcare management as a fellow in the American College of Healthcare Executives (FACHE). His 35 years of healthcare executive experience spans all facets of ambulatory services, including development and operations of community-based primary and multispecialty physician practices, hospital-based ambulatory and faculty practices organizations, quality, and patient safety improvement activities.

Dr. Bittle is the program director for the Master of Health Administration and the innovative online Master of Applied Science in Population Health Management at the Bloomberg School of Public Health. He teaches courses in leadership and management, collective impact and collaboration, healthcare financing, medical practice management, and healthcare strategy. His areas of research interest include physician leadership development, organizational and management factors that influence physician alignment, managing change in complex organizations, and developing effective strategies for collaboration within population health management.

Dr. Bittle earned his Doctorate in Public Health (DrPH), with a concentration in leadership and management, from Johns Hopkins Bloomberg School of Public Health; his MBA from the University of Baltimore; and his Bachelor of Science in Emergency Health Services from the University of Maryland, Baltimore County.

THE WELL-MANAGED AMBULATORY PRACTICE

Elizabeth W. Woodcock, DrPH, MBA, FACMPE, CPC

Mark J. Bittle, DrPH, MBA, FACHE

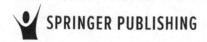

Copyright © 2022 Springer Publishing Company, LLC
All rights reserved.

No part of this publication may be reproduced, stored in a retrieval system, or transmitted in any form or by any means, electronic, mechanical, photocopying, recording, or otherwise, without the prior permission of Springer Publishing Company, LLC, or authorization through payment of the appropriate fees to the Copyright Clearance Center, Inc., 222 Rosewood Drive, Danvers, MA 01923, 978-750-8400, fax 978-646-8600, info@copyright.com or at www.copyright.com.

Springer Publishing Company, LLC
11 West 42nd Street, New York, NY 10036
www.springerpub.com
connect.springerpub.com/

Acquisitions Editor: David D'Addona
Compositor: Amnet Systems

ISBN: 978-0-8261-5662-4
ebook ISBN: 978-0-8261-5663-1
DOI: 10.1891/9780826156631

SUPPLEMENTS:
Instructor materials:

A robust set of instructor resources designed to supplement this text is located at **http://connect.springerpub.com/978-0-8261-5663-1.** Qualifying instructors may request access by emailing **textbook@springerpub.com.**

Instructor's Manual ISBN: **978-0-8261-5664-8**
Instructor Test Bank ISBN: **978-0-8261-5666-5**
Instructor PowerPoints ISBN: **978-0-8261-5665-5**

21 22 23 24 / 5 4 3 2 1

The author and the publisher of this Work have made every effort to use sources believed to be reliable to provide information that is accurate and compatible with the standards generally accepted at the time of publication. The author and publisher shall not be liable for any special, consequential, or exemplary damages resulting, in whole or in part, from the readers' use of, or reliance on, the information contained in this book. The publisher has no responsibility for the persistence or accuracy of URLs for external or third-party Internet websites referred to in this publication and does not guarantee that any content on such websites is, or will remain, accurate or appropriate.

Library of Congress Cataloging-in-Publication Data

Names: Woodcock, Elizabeth W. author. | Bittle, Mark J., author.
Title: The well-managed ambulatory practice / Elizabeth W. Woodcock, Mark
    J. Bittle.
Description: New York, NY : Springer Publishing Company, LLC, [2022] |
    Includes bibliographical references and index.
Identifiers: LCCN 2021035735 (print) | LCCN 2021035736 (ebook) | ISBN
    9780826156624 (paperback) | ISBN 9780826156631 (ebook)
Subjects: MESH: Practice Management, Medical—organization & administration
    | Ambulatory Care—organization & administration
Classification: LCC RA974 (print) | LCC RA974 (ebook) | NLM W 80 | DDC
    362.12068—dc23
LC record available at https://lccn.loc.gov/2021035735
LC ebook record available at https://lccn.loc.gov/2021035736

Contact sales@springerpub.com to receive discount rates on bulk purchases.

Publisher's Note: New and used products purchased from third-party sellers are not guaranteed for quality, authenticity, or access to any included digital components.

Printed in the United States of America.

This book is dedicated to Deborah Walker Keegan, PhD, FACMPE, MBA, who made significant contributions to the field of practice management. Her experience and expertise have left an indelible mark on the many practices with which she worked—and the myriad physician and administrative leaders who learned from her engaging and informative presentations. Deborah always approached her work with an academic rigor, bringing scholar and professionalism to a field that had historically relied on instinct and intuition. Deborah's thirst for knowledge, her passion for improvement, and her focus on evidence-based practices were unparalleled, and the field of practice management is far better because of her. It is an honor to dedicate this book to Deborah to further her goal of guiding, enlightening, and educating the leaders of ambulatory practices.

CONTENTS

Contributors   ix
Foreword   David C. Chin, MD, MBA   xi
Preface   xiii
Acknowledgments   xv

1. **The Ambulatory Landscape**   1

2. **Strategy and Leadership**   33
   With Contributing Author Jalana McCasland

3. **Organizational Structure**   57
   Carol K. Lucas

4. **Quality, Safety, and Patient Experience**   77
   With Contributing Author Kristin Baird

5. **Operations**   109
   Case Study: Lemonaid Health: Pursuing a New Strategy in Mental Health   146

6. **Financial Management**   163

7. **Human Resources**   199
   Case Study: Disruptive Behavior by Iris Grimm   223

Acronyms   227
Glossary   231
Index   235

CONTRIBUTORS

Kristin Baird, MHA, BSN, RN, President and CEO, Baird Group, Fort Atkinson, Wisconsin

Rick Evans, Senior Vice President, Patient Services and Chief Experience Officer, New York-Presbyterian Hospital, New York, New York

Iris Grimm, Physician and Leadership Coach, Master Performance, Inc., Atlanta, Georgia

Manoj Jain, MD, MPH, Adjunct Professor, Department of Health Policy and Management, Rollins School of Public Health, Emory University, Atlanta, Georgia

Mary Ellen Kellogg, Billing Office Supervisor, Ortho NorthEast, Fort Wayne, Indiana

Carol K. Lucas, JD, Shareholder and Chair of the Health Care Practice, Buchalter, Los Angeles, California

Jalana McCasland, Vice President, Physician Practice Management, Children's Hospital of The King's Daughters, Norfolk, Virginia

Michelle Ossmann, PhD, MSN, Assoc. AIA, Director of Knowledge and Innovation, Herman Miller Healthcare, Zeeland, Michigan

Mona Reimers, MBA, Director of Administrative Operations, Ortho NorthEast, Fort Wayne, Indiana

Concettina (Tina) Tolomeo, DNP, MBA, APRN, FNP-BC, AE-C, Senior Director, Patient Access, Yale Medicine, New Haven, Connecticut

FOREWORD

This first edition of *The Well-Managed Ambulatory Practice* appears at a time when several major forces in the American health system have converged to drive improvement in health and value in this approximately $4 trillion sector of the economy. The affirmation of the Affordable Care Act by the Supreme Court likely makes permanent the expansion of Medicaid. An increase in the insured population not only propels the demand for ambulatory care but also complements the continued efforts by the federal government to move to value-based reimbursement models. The initiatives include managed Medicaid, through which the majority of enrollees receive all or part of their care from risk-based arrangements. When these Medicaid and Medicare enrollees are added to the millions of commercial lives receiving care under the alternative payment models that were created by the Medicare Access and CHIP Reauthorization Act in 2015, one can see that a major shift is underway in provider reimbursement away from fee for service and toward value. The change in incentives has driven the move from inpatient care toward ambulatory care and increased the importance of patient-centered medical homes (PCMH) as a cornerstone to improve health outcomes and reduce costs.

The shift toward ambulatory care has been accelerated by the once-in-a-century COVID-19 pandemic. Access to hospitals and clinics were severely curtailed due to pandemic restrictions, which drove relaxation of regulatory barriers and the movement to telehealth and in-home care out of necessity. Providers have been able to leverage new online video applications, the availability of electronic health records, and broadband internet to expand telehealth. Given consumer expectations of convenience, driven by their experience with other online services, and a continued introduction of novel remote monitoring technologies, the trend toward greater reliance on ambulatory care—in this instance more remote care—will accelerate, reinforced by the more efficient use of providers and demand from patients.

The pandemic also exposed some of the major weaknesses in our system—an atrophied public health infrastructure; health disparities and inequities resulting from the lack of investment in the social determinants of health; and clinician burnout. While better practice management cannot address these issues alone, it will be the cornerstone of any successful strategies to address these important issues.

As a former head of a large prepaid group practice and lead partner of a "Big Four" academic medical center and provider consulting practice, I can see that the authors have distilled their decades of ambulatory practice management experience into pithy and actionable insights. They have provided a clear historical context and delineated how to create a vision and strategy; how to lead the required changes, employing emotional intelligence; and how deploy quality improvement methodologies for performance improvement. They also provide important details on how to improve operations, especially in the critically important areas of PCMH, patient flow and access, revenue cycle and financial management, and human resource management with specific guidance on optimal staffing ratios.

This textbook benefits from the accumulated wisdom of two very accomplished healthcare leaders. Elizabeth Woodcock is the founder of the Patient Access Collaborative, which is a group of 90 academic healthcare delivery systems working to promulgate industry standards for patient access. She has authored 17 books, including several on patient flow, front office management, and a policies and procedures for medical practices. Her published works draw on her experiences as a former administrator of the business office for a 500-physician medical group, a longtime consultant for the Medical Group Management Association, and a passionate advocate for better patient access.

Mark Bittle is the director of the Johns Hopkins Bloomberg School of Public Health Master of Health Administration and the Master of Applied Science in Population Health Management programs. As a fellow faculty member in the Department of Health Policy and Management, I have had the privilege of collaborating with him over the years in these programs. His major academic interests include physician leadership development, organizational alignment of physicians, managing change in complex healthcare organizations, and effective, collaborative strategies to improve population health. He brings decades of senior management experience at Johns Hopkins Medicine and LifeBridge Health. Mark's service to healthcare includes board roles for organizations such as the Maryland Rural Health Association and the Shepherd's Clinic, a unique not-for-profit organization providing free, high-quality care to the uninsured in Baltimore, as governing councilor for the American Public Health Association, and as Regent in the American College of Health Executives for Maryland.

Students of healthcare management and early careerists across the health professions will benefit from this clear and actionable guide to managing and improving ambulatory practice for value and quality in this rapidly evolving and challenging environment.

David C. Chin, MD, MBA
Distinguished Scholar
Department of Health Policy and Management
Johns Hopkins Bloomberg School of Public Health
Baltimore, Maryland

PREFACE

The ambulatory practice is the backbone of the United States healthcare system. Ambulatory practices exist in many forms—from solo, private, family medicine practices to the multispecialty, outpatient clinic enterprise of a large health system. The ambulatory practice offers many opportunities to enhance the care delivery process. Two of the more fundamental opportunities, which in the current environment are of import for future healthcare leaders, include cost and convenience.

An ambulatory practice can be structured to provide high-quality healthcare services with much reduced overhead from the traditional inpatient setting. The ambulatory practice setting is cost-effective, aligning well with one of the goals of the Triple Aim of lowering per capita expenditures, thus creating an opportunity for societal benefit. Ambulatory care provides patients with choice and convenience given the ability to locate services proximate to patient demand. These qualities of the ambulatory practice among the others described in this book require a fundamentally different approach to management compared to the inpatient setting. As value-based reimbursement propels services to the lowest cost settings and patients' expectations for convenient, accessible, affordable healthcare rise, a well-managed ambulatory practice is a necessary and vital component of an effective and efficient healthcare delivery system.

The purpose of this book is to provide current and future leaders with a thorough understanding of the foundations of a well-managed ambulatory practice. Commencing with the storied history of ambulatory care in the United States, *The Well-Managed Ambulatory Practice* takes readers on an evidence-informed journey designed to expand their knowledge about the unique aspects of ambulatory practice personnel; finances; quality, safety, and experience; organization; strategy; and operations. With the accelerating pace of ambulatory practice development and complexity, this book serves as an excellent source of contemporary knowledge and skills specific to leading and managing in the ambulatory setting.

We invite you to learn more about the challenges and opportunities inherent in managing an ambulatory practice.

Elizabeth W. Woodcock, DrPH, MBA, FACMPE, CPC
Mark J. Bittle, DrPH, MBA, FACHE

 A robust set of instructor resources designed to supplement this text is located at http://connect.springerpub.com/978-0-8261-5663-1. Qualifying instructors may request access by emailing textbook@springerpub.com.

ACKNOWLEDGMENTS

We are grateful for Xavier Jones, Amy Shim, and Estelle Woodcock for their myriad contributions to the book. We could not have produced this material without your dedication, attention to detail, and editorial skills. We greatly appreciate the vision and expert guidance of David D'Addona and Jaclyn Shultz of Springer Publishing. Thank you all for your time, support, and contributions to this endeavor.

THE AMBULATORY LANDSCAPE

LEARNING OBJECTIVES

1. Determine the definition of ambulatory practices
2. Understand the history of ambulatory practices in the United States
3. Recognize current and future trends related to ambulatory practices
4. Comprehend the involvement of ambulatory practices in the challenges of the U.S. healthcare delivery system

KEY TERMS

Mobile Health

Patient-Centered

Merger and Acquisition; Consolidation

Population

Rise of Consumerism

Emphasis on Information Technology Interoperability

Shift From Fee-for-Service to Alternative, Value-Based Payment Models

INTRODUCTION

The delivery of ambulatory care in the United States provides an engaging context for management professionals. Management professionals may specialize in ambulatory care as a whole—or dedicate their careers to a single setting within the field. Regardless of the choice, the administration of an ambulatory practice provides a stimulating work environment as it represents a workplace offering a wide spectrum of choices accompanied by a variety of people, processes, and technology. Despite the fluctuating environment, the outcome remains the same: delivering high-quality, service-oriented, cost-effective care to all patients.

DEFINITION

According to the National Center for Health Statistics, *ambulatory medical care* refers to "office visits made by patients to health care providers involved in direct patient care practicing in an office or community health center and customarily including consulting, examination, and/or treatment" (personal correspondence, National Ambulatory Medical Care Staff at the National Center for Health Statistics, March 11, 2021). The term conveys an extensive array of practice settings. The Centers for Disease Control and Prevention (CDC) asserts that ambulatory care settings include community health centers, urgent care centers, retail clinics, hospital-based outpatient clinics, non-hospital-based clinics and physician offices, ambulatory surgical centers, public health clinics, imaging centers, oncology clinics, ambulatory behavioral health and substance abuse clinics, physical therapy, rehabilitation centers, dental offices, school health clinics (college and other), home healthcare, and hospice (nonhospital). The list is not exhaustive; myriad entities are considered ambulatory practices as the definition provides for any entity treating a patient who can ambulate and is not otherwise being managed as an inpatient in a healthcare facility.

Today, the term *ambulatory* is often used interchangeably with *outpatient*, a moniker created to distinguish the setting of care from inpatients who are "in" the hospital. As demonstrated in Table 1.1, the growth of physician and hospital outpatient visits in volume has been substantial; the visit rate per capita has remained steady over time for physician office visits, although increasing for hospital outpatient visits during the same period. New settings, sites, and locations are being constantly added in concert with the ever-changing systems for care delivery, leading to an exciting environment for persons in the field of ambulatory practice management.

Managers working in an ambulatory practice in any setting evidence a wide array of skills and competencies. Those selected by the Medical Group Management Association (MGMA, 2021) as a domain in the body of knowledge for medical practice management, which closely aligns with ambulatory practices, include financial management, human resource management, organizational governance, operations management, risk and compliance management, and transformative healthcare delivery. Ambulatory practice management is valued by physicians, hospitals, community health centers, and public health departments, all of which require skills and expertise in this setting.

HISTORICAL CONTEXT

The evolution of ambulatory care in the United States offers a lens into the complexity of healthcare in the present day. Like many other fields, the history of ambulatory care is weaved into the international context. In the 17th century, physicians in major urban centers in Europe created consultation centers to serve the poor (Sand, 1952). These centers, which were housed in separate facilities from the hospital, provided treatment and medicine to patients not in need of inpatient care. Because medications were dispensed in the consultation centers, they become known as

TABLE 1.1 Annual Physician Office and Hospital Outpatient Visits in the United States, 1973–2016

YEAR	PHYSICIAN OFFICE VISITS[a] (MILLIONS)	PHYSICIAN OFFICE VISIT RATE (PER PERSON)	HOSPITAL OUTPATIENT VISITS[b] (THOUSANDS)	HOSPITAL OUTPATIENT VISIT RATE (PER 100 PERSONS)
1973	644.9	3.1		
1974	577.8	–		
1975	567.6	2.7		
1976	588.3	2.8		
1977	570	2.7		
1978	584.5	2.8		
1979	556.3	2.6		
1980	575.7	2.7		
1981	585.2	2.6		
1982				
1983				
1984				
1985	636.4	2.7		
1986				
1987				
1988				
1989	692.7	2.8		
1990	704.6	2.9		
1991	669.7	2.7		
1992	762	3	56.6	22.5
1993	717.2	2.8	62.5	24.6
1994	681.5	2.6	66.3	25.6
1995	697.1	2.7	67.2	25.7
1996	734.5	2.8	67.2	25.4
1997	787.4	3.0	77.0	28.9
1998	829.3	3.1	75.4	28
1999	756.7	2.785	84.6	31.1

(continued)

TABLE 1.1 (*Continued*)

YEAR	PHYSICIAN OFFICE VISITS[a] (MILLIONS)	PHYSICIAN OFFICE VISIT RATE (PER PERSON)	HOSPITAL OUTPATIENT VISITS[b] (THOUSANDS)	HOSPITAL OUTPATIENT VISIT RATE (PER 100 PERSONS)
2000	823.5	3.004	83.3	30.4
2001	880.5	3.144	83.7	29.9
2002	890	3.144	83.3	29.4
2003	906	3.173	94.6	33.1
2004	910.9	3.159	85	29.5
2005	963.6	3.31	90.4	31
2006	902	3.066	102.2	34.7
2007	994.3	3.356	88.9	30
2008	956.0	3.201	109.9	36.8
2009	1037.8	3.441	96.1	31.9
2010	1008.8	3.322	100.7	33.2
2011	987.0	3.222	125.7	41
2012	928.6	3.008	–	–
2013	922.6	2.967	–	–
2014	884.7	2.8	–	–
2015	990.8	3.133	–	–
2016	883.7	2.779	–	–

SOURCE: National Ambulatory Medical Care Survey (NAMCS)/National Hospital Ambulatory Medical Care Survey (NHAMCS) data were retrieved from summary reports published here: Centers for Disease Control and Prevention, National Center for Health Statistics. (n.d.). *Advance data from vital and health statistics*. https://www.cdc.gov/nchs/products/ad.htm. All material appearing in this report is in the public domain.

NOTE: Physician office visit data retrieved from the NAMCS conducted annually beginning 1973; hospital outpatient visit data retrieved from the NHAMCS conducted annually beginning 1992; NHAMCS data from 2012 to 2016 not released due to quality assurance issues.
[a]Includes patient visits to nonfederal, office-based physicians
[b]Includes patient visits to outpatient departments of nonfederal, short-stay hospitals

"dispensaries." This model—and the name—was replicated in colonial America in the late 18th century (Davis & Warner, 1918).

In the decades that followed, these centers were joined by clinics established by the hospitals that were being erected in urban centers in the newly formed United States of America. Attached to the hospital, the clinics were often referred to as outpatient departments (OPDs). Patients inside the hospital were described as inpatients; patients managed outside of the hospital were outpatients.

The management of public health rose to importance in the 1800s, as evidenced by reports such as that issued in 1850 by Lemuel Shattuck, a Massachusetts-based bookseller and statistician. Shattuck's *Report of the Sanitary Commission of the State of Massachusetts* revealed the importance of public health: "Even those persons who attempted to maintain clean and decent homes were foiled in their efforts to resist diseases if the behavior of others invited the visitation of epidemics" (Rosenkrantz, 1972).

In the United States, both dispensaries and outpatient clinics proliferated during the surge of immigrants in the early 1900s with the primary mission of serving the poor (Davis, 1927). By 1916, 495 hospitals had launched outpatient clinics (Roemer, 1981). The dispensaries were generally operated by physicians; the clinics were controlled by the hospitals. Although not formally, these clinics were also referred to as indigent clinics, a title that stuck for some entities in the United States throughout most of the century.

By 1900, 40 states and several local areas had formed health departments (Institute of Medicine [IOM] Committee for the Study of the Future of Public Health, 1988). In addition to focusing on biomedical advances, the health department's role was to address the root causes of diseases related to sanitation and nutrition (e.g., typhoid and goiter, respectively), poor maternal and infant health, and unsafe working conditions (CDC, 1999). The newly established health departments also provided care to the poor, who were disproportionately impacted by disease. By 1915, there were more than 500 tuberculosis clinics and 500 baby clinics in the United States, mainly operated by city health departments (IOM Committee for the Study of the Future of Public Health, 1988). Patients with financial means, in contrast, sought care directly from private physicians (Roemer, 1971).

The Introduction of Health Insurance

Social insurance was introduced in many industrialized countries across the world, providing the working population the opportunity to see private physicians. A landscape of healthcare delivery that bifurcated patients based on financial means formed near the turn of the century in the United States, with employers offering healthcare to workers—or insurance to obtain it. The railroad companies, some of which employed physicians to treat their workers on-site, introduced prepaid medical care in the late 1880s; by 1930, nearly two million Americans were covered by some type of prepayment arrangement (Reed, 1965). Originally structured as a prepayment plan, Blue Cross Blue Shield commenced during the latter part of this period, expanding insurance to more of the working population.

In contrast to general practitioners, who operated within and served a local community, specialists were typically clustered in hospital OPDs, often in urban centers that served as a geographic hub for a populated area. Given the stigma of the dispensaries and outpatient departments as having association with the treatment of the poor, insurance funds began to organize centers for ambulatory care called polyclinics. In many countries, these sites were funded or affiliated with the government. In the United States, private physicians began to develop ambulatory sites on their own. The Mayo brothers—William and Charles—debuted their dedicated outpatient clinic in Minnesota in 1914, introducing the concept of coordinated care with multiple specialists surrounded by a team of support staff (Fye, 2016).

As the 20th century commenced, dispensaries began to close in the United States due to the new regulations driven by the 1910 Flexner Report and similar efforts to formalize medical training and licensure (Berliner, 1975). Some dispensaries were converted to charitable clinics while others simply closed. The care of the poor was relegated to these charitable clinics or the hospitals that operated outpatient clinics. With a few exceptions, these entities received neither government funding nor payment from patients, although they had become a key component of the training ground for those studying medicine (Ehlke, 2018).

Health departments continued to serve a significant role in ambulatory care, boosted by the development of a federal infrastructure for public health in 1912 when the U.S. Public Health Service was formed (IOM Committee for the Study of the Future of Public Health, 1988). Although there was no blueprint for the services provided, local, county, and state health departments played a significant role in the treatment of communicable diseases, mental health, and maternal and child health.

Within the coming decades, group practices, as they came to be known, proliferated across the United States, launching a new healthcare delivery system, as well as a novel opportunity for management professionals. Americans who were insured—nearly 70% of Americans held hospital insurance by 1960 (Cohen et al., 2009)—increasingly sought care through these group practices. Between 1955 and 1965, the use of outpatient services rose by a remarkable 73% (University of Michigan, 1968). In 1970, only 15% of ambulatory visits were performed at a hospital (Murnaghan, 1973).

In the group practice setting, administrators were drawn to the burgeoning field of medical practice management. The National Association of Clinic Managers first assembled in 1926, later becoming the Medical Group Management Association (MGMA). The American Medical Group Association (AMGA) (n.d.) began in 1950 as the American Association of Medical Clinics, to elevate standards of practice in medical clinics, among other goals. Depending on the specialty, much of the care delivered to patients by group practices was in the ambulatory setting. Medical practice managers, therefore, enhanced their expertise in ambulatory care.

During the same period that group practices were expanding, funding by the federal government was infused into building more hospitals. Grants to the states for hospital construction were issued through the Hill–Burton program, which started via the Hospital Services and Construction Act of 1946 but offered support for years beyond (Berkowitz, 2005). While the majority of Americans were insured, health coverage was limited to hospital and surgical services.

The new financing to hospitals in the United States did not generally benefit the outpatient departments. The lack of reimbursement for outpatient care provided by hospitals adversely impacted the clinics by the mid-century. Indeed, as group practices served those with financial means, outpatient clinics had evolved into care sites almost exclusively for the poor. J. H. Knowles, the director of Boston, Massachusetts–based Massachusetts General Hospital, wrote in 1965: "Turning to the outpatient department of the urban hospital, we find the stepchild of the institution. Traditionally, this has been the least popular area in which to work, and as a result, few advances in medical care and teaching have been harvested here for the benefit of the community" (p. 68). Management of the outpatient hospital clinic lagged as well; "medical administrators . . . are naturally comfortable in the traditional, financially rewarding hospital setting" (Crowley & Riordan, 1988).

In the role of the so-called stepchild, patient service also suffered. In 1966, Dr. John Deitrick, the dean of Cornell University Medical Center, wrote: "For the patient, there are long waiting periods and delays . . . the OPD [outpatient department] does seem to be designed for the convenience of the administration of the hospital . . . there is considerable disregard for the comfort and convenience of the patient and for the efficient and effective use for the physician's time" (p. 65).

Neighborhood health clinics also provided care for the poor; like the hospitals' outpatient clinics, there was no formal funding source or patient care revenue (Ehlke, 2018). Many were erected by volunteers or advocacy organizations, often aimed to address a particular health need or ethnic cohort. Health departments continued to expand at the local, county, and state levels in the United States; although as diverse as the patients they attended, most incorporated the essential function of providing vaccinations to the communities they served (CDC, 1999).

Engagement of U.S. Government

As the delivery system was evolving, coverage for health expenditures was changing too. Healthcare disbursements provided by insurance companies—referred to as third-party payments—provided 49% of personal healthcare expenditures in 1964 (Reed & Hanft, 1966). The passage of the Social Security Amendments of 1965 introduced Medicare and Medicaid the following year, moving the majority of payments to healthcare providers into some form of third-party coverage arrangement by the end of the decade. In addition to hospital insurance, the mid-decade law offered the ability for Americans 65 years and older to purchase insurance that covered physicians' services (Social Security Administration [SSA], n.d.). Accordingly, insurance coverage in the private sector also expanded to incorporate nonhospital services.

Although overshadowed by the adoption of these government insurance programs, the Office of Economic Opportunity (OEO) launched an important initiative in 1965 to fund neighborhood health clinics. Sites designed to provide ambulatory care to specific communities had been launched by various private and public organizations since the turn of the century; however, the OEO's efforts formalized a funding mechanism for these community-based efforts. This infusion of financial support commenced efforts to ramp up community-based ambulatory care, including centers aimed at serving migrants, homeless persons, and residents of public housing; rural health clinics (RHCs) were subsequently designated in 1977 (Taylor, 2004). The National Health Service Corps Program, created in 1970, provided federal funding and support to assign physicians to render care to persons in underserved areas (Heisler, 2018).

Medicare and Medicaid coverage, accompanied by increased funding for medical training, shifted the emphasis back on hospital outpatient clinics in the ensuing years. Once operated on a charitable basis, hospitals began to receive reimbursement for care provided in the outpatient clinic through these government programs, at rates higher than the privately operated group practices (Regenstreif, 1977). Recognizing the importance of the outpatient clinic, momentum led to efforts to address the well-documented problems related to service and efficiency in outpatient clinics after many years of suffering from the lack of economic, public, and professional support in the outpatient setting as compared to the hospital (Stoeckle et al., 1979).

In concert with changes to the delivery system, medical training programs began to shift their focus to the ambulatory setting, staffing students and residents into hospital outpatient clinics as routine shifts essential to their program requirements as learners and trainees, respectively. Educational institutions recognized the importance of longitudinal and comprehensive care for medical students and trainees, best studied in the outpatient setting (Crowley & Riordan, 1988).

There was a growing recognition of the importance of centering care around the patient. The first ambulatory surgery center (ASC) was erected in 1970 and endorsed by the American Medical Association the following year. ASCs proliferated in the 1970s as the model proved successful in addressing challenges of the existing healthcare delivery system related to cost, timeliness, convenience, quality assurance, and comfort (Ambulatory Surgery Center Association, n.d.; Frakes, 2002).

Insurance expanded to cover physician services, and Americans responded with enthusiasm: Between 1970 and 1976, the proportion of the population younger than 65 years with third-party insurance coverage for physician office and home visits increased from 48.0% to 62.2% (Carroll, 1978; Mueller, 1972). Health maintenance organizations (HMOs) were added to the landscape in 1973 upon the passage of the HMO Act, offering a combination of medical care and insurance.

In recognition of the growing importance of the ambulatory setting, the federal government began the National Ambulatory Medical Care Survey (NAMCS) in 1973, a data repository that continues through today. The NAMCS and the National Hospital Ambulatory Medical Care Survey (NHAMCS) provide a consistent source of data about the ambulatory setting, allowing government officials, as well as industry stakeholders, to understand the trends related to ambulatory care.

Skyrocketing Costs in the United States

The shift in reimbursement, designated funding for community health, increased numbers of medical learners and trainees, enhanced by the influence of an aging population and new technology, combined to foster the continued development of ambulatory sites across all settings in the final quarter of the 20th century.

The big story, however, was the massive increase in costs: healthcare spending more than tripled between 1971 and 1981, substantially outpacing economic growth (Freeland & Schendler, 1983). Addressing the rising cost of healthcare in the United States became a critical mission for legislators.

In 1983, prospective payments for hospital services were introduced through diagnosis-related groups (DRGs), followed by a similar payment system for outpatient clinics in 1989 (Mayes, 2007; Oberlander, 2003). Researchers have concluded that these payment systems propelled care to the ambulatory setting (Roos & Freeman, 1989).

The federal government created the Federally Qualified Health Center (FQHC) program in 1989, into which a multitude of neighborhood centers that dated back to the early 1900s evolved. During the same period, the IOM Committee for the Study of the Future of Public Health (1988) issued a report, *The Future of Public Health*, advocating that local health departments concentrate on three essential functions: assessment, policy development, and assurance. Some morphed their service offerings into FQHCs or RHCs; others transferred their health services to hospitals to manage in their outpatient clinics; some narrowed their services to immunizations (Keane et al., 2001).

Other ambulatory sites—school clinics, dialysis centers, infusion centers, urgent care clinics, retail-based clinics, and countless more—were created or expanded their services in the 1990s as patient care increasingly moved away from the acute hospital setting.

Concerned by the growing expenditures for physician services paid on a percent-of-charge basis, the federal government migrated to a new payment system founded on the resource-based relative value scale (RBRVS) in 1993 (Hsiao et al., 1993). This new payment system had a significant impact on ambulatory practices, as it represented the mechanism to reimburse the services of physicians and other healthcare professionals. The RBRVS, a payment system constructed on the components of work, malpractice, and practice expense tied to each procedure code used for professional services, was subsequently adopted by many private insurance companies.

To combat rising costs and utilization, managed care was introduced during this same period. *Managed care*—a term that encompasses a variety of payment mechanisms, notably capitation, linked to administrative functions designed to manage *costs*—created many administrative barriers to accessing care largely focused on the ambulatory setting. Patients were required to obtain authorizations, referrals, and other permissions to be seen by specialists, obtain medications, or have tests performed. The responsibility for acquiring these approvals typically fell on the practice; without them, the patient's insurer would not pay. Because every insurance company had its own take on managed care, administering these processes on behalf of patients was challenging.

In addition to the approval requirements, capitation was adopted as a primary payment method. For participating primary care providers, insurers paid a per-member per-month fee. Specialists were paid under subcapitation or highly discounted fee-for-service arrangements and referrals to the specialists in the network were tightly controlled by the primary care physicians. In general, large, multispecialty group practices with sophisticated administrative infrastructures and the ability to coordinate care across specialties fared better. Despite some gains in controlling costs, managed care was largely rejected by stakeholders—physicians, hospitals, and patients alike—by the turn of the century due to what patients and providers believed to be burdensome and harmful restrictions (Dudley & Luft, 2001; Robinson, 2001).

CURRENT LANDSCAPE

The voice of the consumer grew louder during the final quarter of the 20th century, driven in part by the financial responsibility increasingly borne by patients for their healthcare (Brook et al., 1984). After the managed care models of the 1990s were rebuffed, insurance returned to a fee-for-service construct at the turn of the century, albeit with the patient carrying a larger portion of the bill. Despite shifting the payment burden to the consumer, the cost of healthcare in the United States continued to rise. Ambulatory practices offer a low-cost setting for care delivery, thus enhancing the prominence of these settings in the U.S. healthcare system as a means to address growing expectations for the best care at the lowest cost. Technology innovations have permitted more advanced levels of care to be shifted from the traditional hospital-based setting into ambulatory care facilities, thus increasing the demand for ambulatory sites of care delivery. Insurers also have modified fee schedules for a growing list of ambulatory-only procedures in which the provider will only be paid if the care was provided in the ambulatory setting.

Delivery Systems

The healthcare infrastructure in the United States is evolving to face today's challenges. Key stakeholders in the U.S. healthcare delivery system as it relates to the settings where ambulatory care is provided include physician offices, hospital outpatient departments, community health centers, and public health departments.

Physician Offices

Physicians practice in a multitude of settings in the United States. Physician groups, most of which are housed in an office-based ambulatory practice, may be single or multispecialty. The physician may have a single office suite, or the office may be supplemented by other ambulatory sites of care. For example, a gastroenterology practice may have an office with exam rooms and an endoscopy suite; a multispecialty practice may provide a full complement of primary, medical, and surgical specialties, each with corresponding facilities that feature ambulatory practices with office spaces, procedure rooms, infusion suites, ambulatory surgery centers, and so forth. Physician groups may operate as independent businesses. Alternatively, these entities may merge or affiliate with practices in their community or develop similar relationships outside of the local market to form what is commonly called a "supergroup" on a regional or national scale.

Physician employment is on the rise. In contrast to the independent, physician-owned model of ambulatory practice that dominated the better part of the 20th century in the United States, 42% of physicians were employed by hospitals in July 2016, compared to one in four physicians in July 2012 (see Figure 1.1). In 2020,

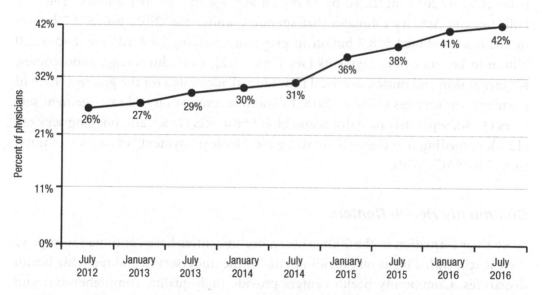

FIGURE 1.1 Percentage of hospital-employed physicians in the United States, 2012–2016.

SOURCE: Physician Advocacy Institute. (2017). *Latest PAI research efforts.* http://www.physiciansadvocacyinstitute.org/PAI-Research/Physician-Employment-Physician. Practice Acquisition Study: National and Regional Employment Changes.

NOTE: Avalere analysis of SK&A hospital/health system ownership of physician practice locations data with Medicare 5% Standard Analytic Files.

In July 2016, the total number of physicians decreased. As a result, the number of employed physicians decreased slightly but the percentage of employed physicians increased.

50.2% of practicing physicians were employed, while 44% owned their practices, according to the Physician Practice Benchmark Survey by the American Medical Association (2021).

Hospital Outpatient Departments

Hospitals and health systems are growing their OPDs, which have retained the ability to achieve a higher fee structure than providers operating in the physicians' office setting. The hospital-based outpatient departments—often referred to as outpatient clinics—are reimbursed under the Outpatient Prospective Payment System (OPPS), a separate fee schedule that is updated annually by the hospital market basket index less a multifactor productivity adjustment. Table 1.2 illustrates the growth in outpatient utilization for outpatient clinic visits, as well as outpatient surgeries in community hospitals.

According to the Centers for Medicare and Medicaid Services (CMS, 2020), 96% of the nation's nearly 3,300 acute care hospitals provided outpatient services in 2018, up from 94% in 2008. Data regarding spending on hospital outpatient services by Medicare demonstrate increased spending. Overall spending by Medicare and beneficiaries on hospital outpatient services covered under the OPPS from 2009 to 2019 increased by 114%, an average of 7.9% per annum. The U.S. Office of the Actuary estimates that spending under the OPPS was $72.7 billion in 2019, a combined $58.7 billion in program spending by Medicare, and $14.0 billion in beneficiary copayments (see Figure 1.2). Procedures (e.g., endoscopies, surgeries, skin and musculoskeletal procedures) accounted for the greatest share of payments for services (47%) in 2018, followed by evaluation and management services (19%), separately paid drugs and blood products (18%), and imaging services (12%), according to a claims analysis by the Medical Payment Advisory Commission (MedPAC, 2020).

Community Health Centers

Since their formation in the 20th century, health centers have continued to expand their reach, with a focus on providing care for the underserved and reducing health disparities. Community health centers provide high-quality, comprehensive, and affordable primary care to medically underserved patients, regardless of their ability to pay (National Association of Community Health Centers, 2021). Of the patients served by health centers in 2019, 91% were in or near poverty, as measured by the National Association of Community Health Centers. Consistent with the overall growth in ambulatory visit volume since the turn of the 21st century, similar trends are demonstrated by the increase in health center patients and visits between 2009 and 2019 (see Figure 1.3).

TABLE 1.2 Outpatient Utilization in Community Hospitals, 1995–2018

YEAR	TOTAL OUTPATIENT VISITS	OUTPATIENT VISITS PER 1,000	OUTPATIENT SURGERIES
1995	413,748,403	1,574.6	13,462,304
1996	439,863,107	1,658.3	14,023,651
1997	450,140,010	1,681.9	14,678,290
1998	474,193,468	1,756.3	15,593,614
1999	495,346,286	1,816.5	15,845,492
2000	521,404,976	1,852.8	16,383,374
2001	538,480,378	1,890.8	16,684,726
2002	556,404,212	1,931.1	17,361,176
2003	563,186,046	1,936.7	17,165,616
2004	571,569,334	1,946.4	17,351,490
2005	590,588,050	2,002 0	17,914,688
2006	605,360,605	2,031.4	17,759,341
2007	609,950,981	2,026.4	17,668,632
2008	632,642,025	2,081.1	17,912,834
2009	648,718,968	2,120.0	17,878,784
2010	659,120,335	2,133.1	17,947,041
2011	663,014,495	2,131.9	17,796,0M
2012	681,543,152	2,177.5	17,819,454
2013	684,227,319	2,165.3	17,978,474
2014	700,231,991	2,202.0	17,974,397
2015	730,789,365	2,283.7	18,255,921
2016	756,797,776	2,343.0	18,987,342
2017	766,076,124	2,357.2	19,075,759
2018	766,390,000	2,336.6	19,168,038

SOURCE: Analysis of American Hospital Association Annual Survey data, 2018, for community hospitals. US Census Bureau. (2018, July 1). *National and State Population Estimates.* https://www.census.gov/data/tables/time-series/demo/popest/2010s-national-detail.html. Data for Charts 3.9, 3.10 and 3.11; https://www.aha.org/system/files/media/file/2020/10/TrendwatchChartbook-2020-Appendix.pdf.

Public Health Departments

Public health departments engage in ambulatory practice to address community needs at the local, state, territorial, and national levels (see Exhibit 1.1). Public

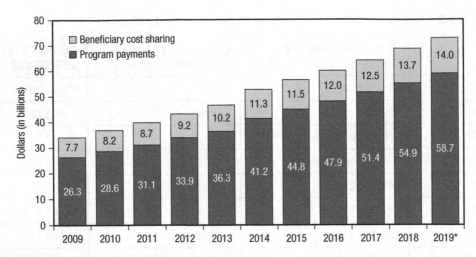

FIGURE 1.2 Medicare spending on hospital outpatient services.

SOURCE: Medical Payment Advisory Commission. (2020, July). *Section 7: Ambulatory care. A data book: Health care spending and the medicare program* (p. 89). http://www.medpac.gov/docs/default-source/data-book/july2020 _databook_sec7_sec.pdf?sfvrsn=0

NOTE: PPS, prospective payment system. Spending amounts are for services covered by the Medicare outpatient PPS. They do not include services paid on separate fee schedules (e.g., ambulance services and durable medical equipment) or those paid on a cost basis (e.g., corneal tissue acquisition, flu vaccines) or payments for clinical laboratory services, except those packaged into payment bundles.
*Estimated figures.

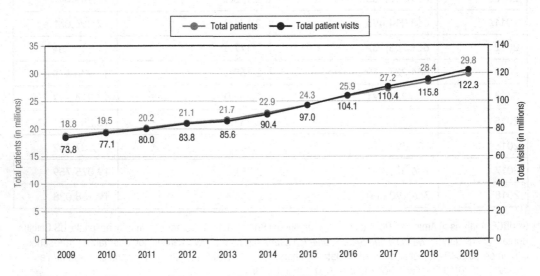

FIGURE 1.3 Health center patients and visits, 2009–2019.

SOURCE: National Association of Community Health Centers. (2021). *Community health center chartbook* (p. 27). https://www.nachc.org/wp-content/uploads/2021/04/Chartbook-Final-2021.pdf

EXHIBIT 1.1 TEN ESSENTIAL PUBLIC HEALTH SERVICES

1. Assess and monitor population health status, factors that influence health, and community needs and assets

2. Investigate, diagnose, and address health problems and hazards affecting the population

3. Communicate effectively to inform and educate people about health, factors that influence it, and how to improve it

4. Strengthen, support, and mobilize communities and partnerships to improve health

5. Create, champion, and implement policies, plans, and laws that impact health

6. Utilize legal and regulatory actions designed to improve and protect the public's health

7. Assure an effective system that enables equitable access to the individual services and care needed to be healthy

8. Build and support a diverse and skilled public health workforce

9. Improve and innovate public health functions through ongoing evaluation, research, and continuous quality improvement

10. Build and maintain a strong organizational infrastructure for public health

SOURCE: Centers for Disease Control and Prevention. (2020). *Ten essential public health services.* https://www.cdc.gov/publichealthgateway/publichealthservices/essentialhealthservices.html.

health departments play a prominent role in not only prevention but also emergency response. For example, with the declaration of the COVID-19 pandemic as a public health emergency in early 2020, health departments nationwide were thrust into the spotlight to monitor COVID-19 case surveillance, detect outbreaks, administer contact tracing efforts, and provide access to necessary testing and vaccination services. With this, public health departments required close communication with hospitals and laboratory services to assess their caseload and monitor the capacity of local hospitals, as well as integrate safety precautions with facility protocols to ensure the safety of healthcare personnel. In their efforts to protect and improve the health of all communities, health departments play an essential role across all healthcare settings, including ambulatory.

Industry Trends

The current landscape is influenced by patients, who are demanding better service and access, at a lower cost. Insisting on more value from the U.S. healthcare system,

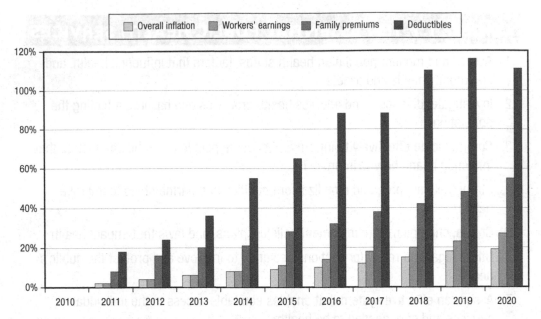

FIGURE 1.4 Employer premiums, deductibles, and wages, 2010–2020.

SOURCE: KFF. (2020, October). *Average family premiums rose 4% to $21,342 in 2020, benchmark KFF employer health benefit survey finds.* https://www.kff.org/health-costs/press-release/average-family-premiums-rose-4-to -21342-in-2020-benchmark-kff-employer-health-benefit-survey-finds/

NOTE: Average general annual deductibles are for single coverage and are among all covered workers. Workers in plans without a general annual deductible for in-network services are assigned a value of zero.

consumers are joined by government officials and insurance companies, who are the largest buyers of healthcare. Trends have emerged as ambulatory practices strive to meet the challenges posed by consumers and purchasers: Patients are engaging in their healthcare; stakeholders are focusing on prevention; value-based payment models are emerging as an alternative to fee-for-service reimbursement; technology is impacting the industry; new organizational structures are being embraced; and access to insurance coverage for all Americans remains a challenge.

Patient Engagement

Patient financial responsibility for health insurance has escalated at a rapid pace since the turn of the century; for employees in the aggregate, the explosive growth outstripped earnings between 2010 and 2020 (see Figure 1.4). Copayments, coinsurance, and deductibles depend on the patient's health plan; however, the framework typically bifurcates benefits for care rendered in the ambulatory setting from the care provided in the hospital. Patients may, therefore, have a separate deductible for the care they receive from an ambulatory practice—and sometimes, there is a further breakdown of the components within an overall deductible scheme.

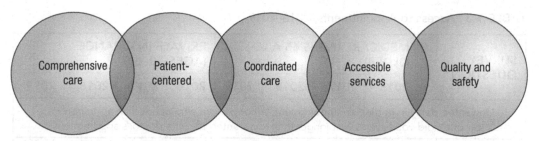

FIGURE 1.5 Patient-centered medical home (PCMH) functions and attributes.

SOURCE: Agency for Healthcare Research and Quality. (n.d.). *Defining the PCMH*. U.S. Department of Health and Human Services. https://pcmh.ahrq.gov/page/defining-pcmh

The financial aspect of healthcare was not the only component of care influenced by patients' participation. There is a recognition that patients should be an integral part of their care and recognized as a member of the care team. **Patient-centered** care models such as the "medical home," a term first coined by pediatricians managing children with complex needs in the 1960s (Sia et al., 2004), have been extended to many ambulatory settings, particularly those delivering primary care. According to the Agency for Healthcare Research and Quality, *medical home* is defined "not simply as a place but as a model of the organization of primary care that delivers the core functions of primary health care" (see Figure 1.5).

As patients engage in their healthcare, their requests for convenience are increasing. This includes timely access to healthcare, a goal echoed by the IOM to ensure the quality of care (IOM Committee on Quality of Health Care in America, 2001; (see Table 1.3, a demonstration of the U.S. government's monitoring of Americans' access to care).

In addition to embracing efforts to reduce appointment wait times, ambulatory practices are addressing this demand in myriad offerings: omnichannel communication platforms; online self-service scheduling, registration, and records access; extended hours of operation; remote monitoring and virtual care; and other innovative strategies.

Preventive Care

The need to stem expenditures in healthcare has exerted more pressure on the industry to find ways not only to manage patients in lower cost settings with timely access but also to focus on prevention. Keeping patients healthy has been a core component of population health, a trend that gained traction at the turn of the 21st century. The National Academy of Medicine (NAM, 2021) purports improvement initiatives to identify and enhance aspects of or contributors to population health, expanding the focus beyond traditional healthcare delivery systems. This holistic view of health has given rise to ambulatory practices playing an integral role in

TABLE 1.3 Access to Appointments, 2016–2019

SURVEY QUESTION	MEDICARE (AGES 65 AND OLDER)				PRIVATE INSURANCE (AGES 50–64)			
	2016	2017	2018	2019	2016	2017	2018	2019
Unwanted delay in getting an appointment: Among those who needed an appointment, "How often did you have to wait longer than you wanted to get a doctor's appointment?"								
FOR ROUTINE CARE								
NEVER	68%[b]	73%[a]	70%[ab]	72%	67%[b]	69%[ab]	64%[ab]	74%
SOMETIMES	22	20[a]	20[a]	20	23[b]	22[ab]	26[ab]	19
USUALLY	4[b]	3	5[b]	3	5	4	5	4
ALWAYS	3	3	3[a]	3	4[b]	3	4[ab]	3
FOR ILLNESS OR INJURY								
NEVER	79[a]	80[a]	79[a]	80	75[ab]	76[ab]	74[ab]	81
SOMETIMES	16[a]	15[a]	15[a]	14	19[ab]	18[ab]	19[ab]	15
USUALLY	2[a]	2	2	2	3[ab]	2	3[b]	2
ALWAYS	2[a]	1[a]	2	2	3[ab]	2[a]	2	1

SOURCE: Medical Payment Advisory Commission. (2020, July). *Section 7: Ambulatory care. A data book: Health care spending and the Medicare program* (p. 84). http://www.medpac.gov/docs/default-source/data-book/july2020_databook_sec7_sec.pdf?sfvrsn=0.

NOTE: Numbers may not sum to 100% due to rounding and to missing responses ("Don't Know" or "Refused") not being presented. Overall sample sizes for each group (Medicare and privately insured) were approximately 4,000 in all years. Sample sizes for Individual questions varied.
[a]Statistically significant difference (at a 95% confidence level) between the Medicare and privately insured samples in the given year.
[b]Statistically significant difference (at a 95% confidence level) from 2019 within the same insurance coverage category

identifying and addressing patients' social determinants of health (SDOH). SDOH, according to the CDC, are "conditions in the places where people live, learn, work, and play that affect a wide range of health and quality-of-life risks and outcomes." See Figure 1.6 for the five key areas of SDOH according to the CDC.

Value-Based Care

The growing focus on the patient has challenged the notion of outcomes—one can quantify revenue and costs, but how do we measure *value*? Is the notion of value built on individual patient outcomes of care received, clinical quality with the absence of significant morbidity, the balance between cost and effectiveness of delivered care, patient service, or some other variable? Value-based care has dominated

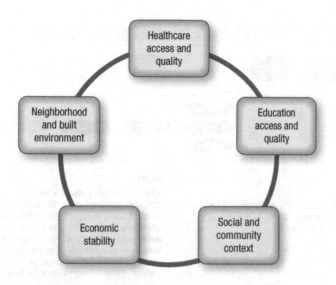

FIGURE 1.6 Five key areas of social determinants of health (SDOH).

SOURCE: Centers for Disease Control and Prevention. (2020, August 19). *Social determinants of health: Know what affects health.* U.S. Department of Health and Human Services. https://www.cdc.gov/socialdeterminants/about.html

the vernacular of industry stakeholders for the better part of the second and third decades of the 21st century, with management experts weighing in on the definition of value-based healthcare (Porter & Teisberg, 2006).

At the heart of value-based care is a focus on improving the quality of care with a growing emphasis on patient outcomes over the structures and processes of care. Defining, measuring, and ultimately improving patient outcomes in the ambulatory setting remains a challenge. The rapid development of ambulatory services and the continued expansion of clinical activities now performed in the various organizational forms that define the ambualtory sector make the integration and coordination of care across the ambualtory sector difficult. Coupled with the challenges of measuring and manging quality in the ambulatory setting is the fact that many value-based care models have been introduced by the government (for Medicare and Medicaid), as well as private insurers. (Figure 1.7 displays the evolution of value-based programs at the federal level.) Although different in construct, the overarching theme is to reward healthcare professionals and facilities for the balanced delivery of high-quality, cost-efficient care. As an integral component of the healthcare delivery system in the United States, ambulatory practices remain front and center in these new models.

Impact of Technology

Although technology has played a role in advancements in ambulatory care for decades, the introduction of the electronic health record (EHR) system resulted in a drastic transformation of people and processes. The growth in EHR system adoption

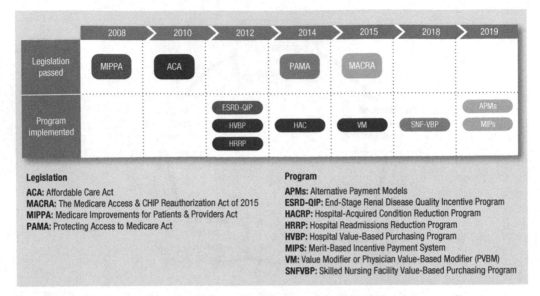

FIGURE 1.7 The evolution of value-based programs at the federal level.

SOURCE: Centers for Medicare and Medicaid Services. (2020, January 6). *CMS' value-based programs.* https://www.cms.gov/Medicare/Quality-Initiatives-Patient-Assessment-Instruments/Value-Based-Programs/ Value-Based-Programs

in the early 21st century was strongly facilitated by the government via the EHR Incentive Program. This was a program borne from the Health Information Technology for Economic and Clinical Health Act, a component of the American Recovery and Reinvestment Act of 2009 (ARRA), which provided incentives to physicians and hospitals to facilitate adoption. Medical record technicians—a key staff support role—gave way to data management experts; rooms previously full of paper medical records were converted into exam rooms or administrative space. These personnel and facility changes were accompanied by a shift in clinical processes made possible through the real-time access to data by ambulatory practices. Everything from phone messages and referrals to how care is delivered has been transformed by the EHR system. The majority of ambulatory practices now rely on EHR systems; Figure 1.8 provides data about adoption by office-based physicians.

Beyond the EHR system, practice management systems that integrate key functions of ambulatory practices such as registration, scheduling, and billing have become ubiquitous. Similarly, technological tools designed to support healthcare prevention and wellness are proliferating—witness the explosion of wearable devices, home monitoring tools, home diagnostic aids, embedded monitors, and other similar innovations to support patients and help them meet their goals. Technology is enabling more opportunities for ambulatory practices; dramatic advances in technology and science have a major impact on the ambulatory setting (Goldfield, 2017).

Ambulatory practices are expending innovative efforts to respond to the increasing demand for convenience, access, and affordability by patients. Efforts are being

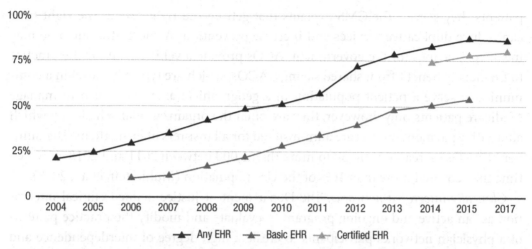

FIGURE 1.8 Electronic health record (EHR) adoption by office-based physicians.

SOURCE: Office of the National Coordinator for Health Information Technology. (2019, January). *Office-based physician electronic health record adoption.* Health IT Quick-Stat #50. https://www.healthit.gov/data/quickstats/office-based-physician-electronic-health-record-adoption

made to streamline access to ambulatory visits by leveraging technology to seamlessly deliver automated self-service scheduling, registration, and records access, among others and deploying natural language processing to enable automated communication and scheduling workflows.

Organizational Structures

Efforts to improve healthcare cannot succeed without the engagement of ambulatory practices, as they are recognized as critical to the success of the healthcare delivery system. Although ever-evolving as rules and regulations shift, an ambulatory practice may be part of one or more of the following organizational structures:

Physician hospital organizations. As ambulatory practices gained prominence, establishments of hospitals and physicians formed relationships. These associations were often formalized as physician–hospital organizations (PHOs); independent practice associations (IPAs) represent a similar model but without a hospital partner. The function of PHOs and IPAs vary significantly; however, many of these organizations serve to contract with insurance companies on behalf of their members. These organizations offer value to participants in such areas as education and training, access to administrative functions, and group purchasing discounts. Considered first-generation relationships, many PHOs and IPAs have evolved involved into more sophisticated models.

Accountable care organizations. According to the CMS, accountable care organizations (ACOs) represent "groups of doctors, hospitals, and other healthcare providers, who come together voluntarily to give coordinated high-quality care to the Medicare patients they serve." The CMS explains that getting the right care at the right time can reduce duplicative services and increase prevention. A successful outcome may mean cost savings for the government; ACOs provide a vehicle to allow the practice to financially benefit from shared savings. ACOs, which are typically based in a community to serve a patient population in a geographical area, may form to manage Medicare patients only; however, they are often the organizational vehicles by which alternative payment models are administered for all insurers offering them. The number of ACOs increased from 58 to more than 1,000 between 2011 and 2018, at which time they covered more than 10% of the U.S. population (Muhlestein et al., 2018).

Clinically integrated networks. The Department of Justice defined clinical integration as "an active and ongoing program to evaluate and modify the practice patterns of a physician network's participants to create a high degree of interdependence and cooperation among the physician members" (Department of Justice and Federal Trade Commission, 1996). Networks, typically aimed at a geographical area, may be formed by leveraging the assets of a hospital or health system; however, they also may be a function of affiliations. Regardless of structure, a clinically integrated network (CIN) uses its collective, integrated resources to provide high-quality, coordinated care. The CIN may contract with insurance companies or directly with employers, perhaps negotiating favorable rates based on demonstrated quality or cost savings for patients served.

Ambulatory practices participate in these evolving organizational structures to engage as a collective group to offer services.

Access to Insurance

Although most Americans are insured, there remain a significant minority of patients who are not. According to most studies, there is a positive relationship between health insurance coverage and health outcomes (IOM Committee on the Consequences of Uninsurance, 2002). Access to insurance coverage is important. The number of uninsured Americans has decreased since the passage of the Affordable Care Act (ACA) from 17.1% in 2008 to 10.4% a decade later (see Figure 1.9).

Although the ACA facilitated access to insurance for some, many of the remaining persons have access to purchase coverage but cite financial constraints as a barrier. In 2019, 73.7% of uninsured adults said that they were uninsured because the cost of coverage was too high, according to the Kaiser Family Foundation (Tolbert et al., 2020). The economic resources of a family may determine access to insurance coverage; Figure 1.10 displays insurance status based on income-to-poverty ratio in addition to other characteristics.

According to researchers at the Commonwealth Fund (Collins & Aboulafia, 2021), other reasons for the lack of insurance include being eligible but not enrolled in Medicaid or the Children's Health Insurance Program (CHIP), existing below the poverty line but living in a Medicaid nonexpansion state, being an undocumented

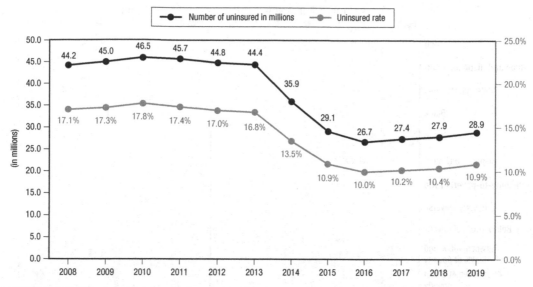

FIGURE 1.9 Number of uninsured and uninsured rate among the nonelderly population, 2008–2019.

SOURCE: Data from KFF analysis of 2008–2019 American Community Survey, 1-Year Estimates. Adapted from Tolbert, J., Orgera, K., & Damico, A. (2020, November). Key facts about the uninsured population. *Kaiser Family Foundation*. https://www.kff.org/uninsured/issue-brief/key-facts-about-the-uninsured-population/.

NOTE: Includes nonelderly individuals ages 0 to 64.

immigrant, and a lack of awareness and barriers to enrolling in low- or no-cost insurance. The cohort of Americans who are not insured remains an important population of patients to be served in communities across the country. Ambulatory practices have and will continue to play a fundamental role in executing this goal.

FUTURE LANDSCAPE

The healthcare delivery system in the United States has been in a state of near-constant change for most, if not all, of the nation's history. There appears to be no end to this state of affairs. The costs associated with healthcare are projected to rise in the United States, yet health outcomes are poor in comparison with other nations. The United States has high rates of chronic diseases, infant mortality, and avoidable deaths (Organisation for Economic Co-operation and Development, 2020). Ambulatory practices will continue to play an important role in combatting cost escalation and poor health outcomes in the U.S. healthcare delivery system.

Cost Escalation

Healthcare costs in the United States have continued to soar, and projections into the future demonstrate no slowdown in growth (see Figure 1.11). Overall, the United States spent $3.8 trillion in healthcare expenditures in 2019, a growth of 4.6% from

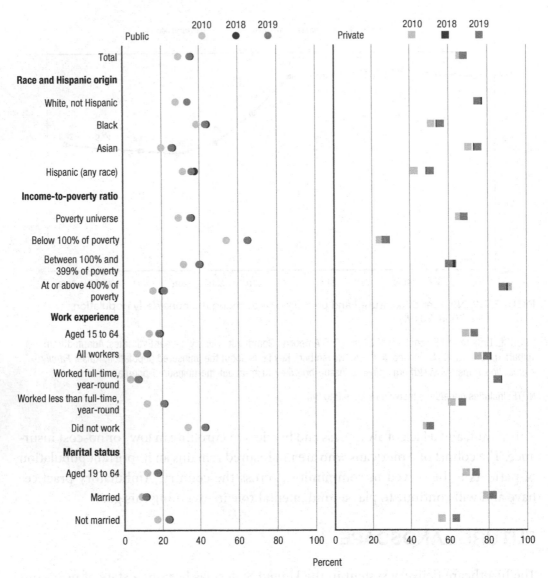

FIGURE 1.10 Insurance coverage expressed in income-to-poverty ratios: 2010, 2018, and 2019.

SOURCE: Keisler-Starkey, K., & Bunch, L. N. (2020). *Health insurance coverage in the United States: 2019* (p. 10). U.S. Government Publishing Office. https://www.census.gov/content/dam/Census/library/publications/2020/demo/p60-271.pdf.

NOTE: Differences are calculated with unrounded numbers, which may produce different results from using the rounded values in the figure. The estimates by type of coverage are not mutually exclusive; people can be covered by more than one type of health insurance during the year. For information on confidentiality protection, sampling error, nonsampling error, and definitions in the American Community Survey, see https://www2.census.gov/programs-surveys/acs/tech_docs/accuracy/ACS_Accuracy_of_Data_2019.pdf.
[1]The poverty universe excludes unrelated individuals younger than 15 years such as foster children.

the prior year, according to the CMS (2020). The federal agency calculated the average healthcare spending per person to equate to $11,582 (CMS, 2020). In terms of its share of the nation's gross domestic product (GDP), healthcare expenditures accounted for 17.7% of GDP in 2019 (CMS, 2020). This rose to 18.0% in 2020,

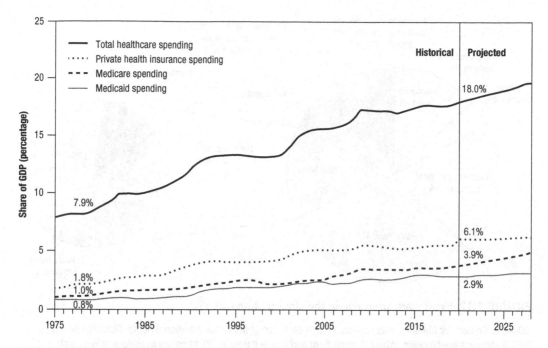

FIGURE 1.11 Healthcare spending as a share of gross domestic product (percentage).

SOURCE: MedPAC analysis of CMS's National Health Expenditure Accounts, historical data released December 2020 and projections released March 2020 as presented in the March 2021 Report to The Congress: Medicare Payment Policy.

NOTE: GDP (gross domestic product). First projected year is 2020. Percentages labeled on the graph are for 1975 and 2020. Beginning in 2014, private health insurance spending includes federal subsidies for both premiums and cost sharing for the health insurance marketplace created by the Affordable Care Act. healthcare spending also includes the following expenditures (not shown): out-of-pocket spending, spending by other health insurance programs (the Children's Health Insurance Program, the Department of Federal Affairs, and the Department of Defense), and other third-party payers and programs and public health activity (including Indian Health Service, Substance Abuse and Mental Health Services Administration, maternal and child health, school health; workers' compensation, work-site healthcare, vocational rehabilitation, and other federal, state, and local programs). The potential effects of the coronavirus pandemic are not reflected in these projections.

according to an analysis conducted by MedPAC. National healthcare expenditures include the annual spending for healthcare goods and services, public health activities, government administration, the net cost of health insurance, and investment related to healthcare.

As demonstrated in Figure 1.12, ambulatory practices are not a distinctly measurable component of the national healthcare expenditures. Indeed, ambulatory practices are nestled in all areas, including physician and clinical services, as well as hospital services (for the sites constructed as hospital outpatient clinics).

Employment

The growth in the demand for ambulatory care is reflected in the employment data. The projections for employment in the ambulatory sector are positive: The Bureau of Labor Statistics (USBLS, 2020) reported 7.7 million Americans employed in ambulatory

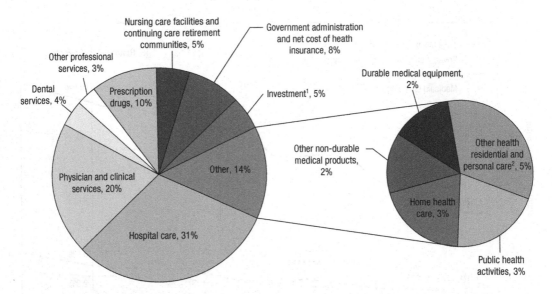

FIGURE 1.12 Healthcare spending in the United States, 2019.

SOURCE: Centers for Medicare and Medicaid Services, Office of the Actuary, National Health Statistics Group. (2020). *Nation's health dollar: Where it came from and where it went* (p. 2). https://www.cms.gov/Research -Statistics-Data-and-Systems/Statistics-Trends-and-Reports/NationalHealthExpendData/NationalHealth AccountsHistorical.

NOTE: Sum of pieces may not equal 100% due to rounding.
[1]Includes work-site healthcare, other private revenues, Indian Health Service, workers' compensation, general assistance, maternal and child health, vocational rehabilitation, Substance Abuse and Mental Health Services Administration, school health, and other federal and state local programs.
[2]Includes copayments, deductibles, and any amounts not covered by health insurance.

TABLE 1.4 Employment and Output in Ambulatory Healthcare Services

EMPLOYMENT							OUTPUT				
THOUSANDS OF JOBS			CHANGE		COMPOUND ANNUAL RATE OF CHANGE		BILLIONS OF CHAINED 2012 DOLLARS			COMPOUND ANNUAL RATE OF CHANGE	
2009	2019	2029	2009–2019	2019–2029	2009–2019	2019–2029	2009	2019	2029	2009–2019	2019–2029
5,793.3	7,697.3	9,124.1	1,904.0	1,426.8	2.9	1.7	811.4	1,086.6	1,457.6	3.0	3.0

SOURCE: United States Bureau of Labor Statistics. (2020, September 1). *Table 2.7: Employment and output by industry.* https://www.bls.gov/emp/tables/industry-employment-and-output.htm.

healthcare services in 2019. The compound annual rate of change projected for 2019 to 2029 is 1.7%, compared to 0.5% for hospitals and 0.4% for all jobs (BLS, 2020). Table 1.4 displays the employment and output data for the ambulatory healthcare services sector.

TABLE 1.5 Encounters per Medicare Beneficiary and Mix of Clinicians

SPECIALTY CATEGORY	ENCOUNTERS PER BENEFICIARY		CHANGE IN ENCOUNTERS PER BENEFICIARY	
	2013	2018	AVERAGE ANNUAL	TOTAL
PRIMARY CARE PHYSICIANS	4.1	3.6	−2.9%	−13.7%
SPECIALISTS	12.5	12.8	0.4%	2.0%
APRNs/PAs	1.3	2.2	11.5%	72.1%
OTHER PRACTITIONERS	2.8	3.3	2.8%	15.1%
TOTAL (ALL CLINICIANS)	20.8	21.9	1.0%	5.0%

SOURCE: Medical Payment Advisory Commission. (2020, July). *Section 7: Ambulatory care. A data book: Health care spending and the medicare program* (p. 83). http://www.medpac.gov/docs/default-source/data-book/july2020 _databook_sec7_sec.pdf?sfvrsn=0.

NOTE: Data were retrieved from MedPAC analysis of the Carrier Standard Analytic File for 100% of beneficiaries and 2019 annual report of the Board of Trustees of the Medicare trust funds.
APRN, advanced practice registered nurse; PA, physician assistant.

The providers who are rendering care are shifting from being physicians to a more diverse mixture of providers. As demonstrated in Table 1.5, which measured the encounters of Medicare patients (beneficiaries aged 65 and older), the utilization of advanced practice providers has risen over time.

Advanced practice providers may include a physician assistant or an advanced practice registered nurse (encompassing the roles of nurse practitioner, certified nurse specialist, certified nurse-midwife, and certified registered nurse anesthetist). The practice of "incident-to" billing—highlighted in Figure 1.13—likely obscures the role that advanced practice providers play. Within guidelines, incident-to billing allows payment of services by an advanced practice provider in a physician's office to be at the full physician rate, as compared to 85% when the advanced practice provider bills independently. In a report to Congress urging the elimination of the billing practice for Medicare, MedPAC estimates that 5% of all evaluation and management office visits billed by physicians were likely performed by an advanced practice registered nurse or physician assistant in 2016 (O'Donnell & Bloniarz, 2018).

Growth

Estimates about the future suggest continued growth in the delivery of ambulatory care. As demonstrated by Figure 1.14, inpatient volumes are expected to be flat, in contrast to growth in ambulatory settings (16% in hospital outpatient department; 25% in ambulatory surgery centers; 17% in physician offices).

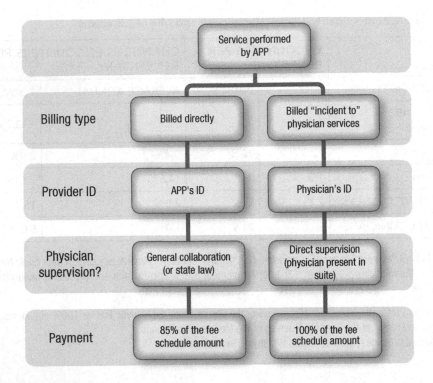

FIGURE 1.13 Structure of incident-to billing.

SOURCE: O'Donnell, B., & Bloniarz, K. (2018). *Medicare payment policies for advanced practice registered nurses and physician assistants*. http://www.medpac.gov/docs/default-source/default-document-library/aprn-pa-slide -deck-final-public.pdf?sfvrsn=0.

APP, advanced practice provider

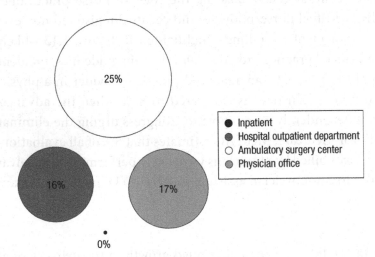

FIGURE 1.14 Procedure forecast by site of care, 2018–2028.

SOURCE: Data from HealthLeaders Fact File (2021, March/April).

HOPD, hospital outpatient department ASC, ambulatory surgery center

The growth in ambulatory volume, combined with the size of the total addressable market of healthcare and the changing expectations of consumers, have attracted many private businesses to healthcare. These include existing companies as well as new entrants. Incumbents, particularly in the retail sector, have invested in opportunities to provide care directly—or support this growing sector. Start-ups have created novel approaches to solve the challenges of the current healthcare system; these young companies are joining existing organizations to render ambulatory care or support the delivery of it. The new approach to care delivery is a key factor in propelling the movement to migrate ambulatory care from traditional office-based practices to computers, mobile devices, and even directly in patients' homes.

CONCLUSION

Based on the historical and projected trajectory of ambulatory care, we can expect new and exciting challenges in this arena for many years to come. As stakeholders aim to ensure healthcare is delivered in the most appropriate and lowest cost setting, the ambulatory care setting will continue to be an indispensable component of the future delivery system as we strive to meet the demand and evolving expectations of patients. The ambulatory setting provides an attractive, challenging, and exciting work environment for managers and leaders who seek a fast-paced, changing environment.

DISCUSSION QUESTIONS

1. The cost of healthcare in the U.S. has risen dramatically. How have ambulatory practices contributed to this rise? How might they be part of the solution?

2. In considering the history of ambulatory practices in the U.S., how did the introduction of insurance alter the landscape? How might the increasing amount of financial responsibility change the environment for ambulatory practices in the future?

3. In your opinion, what is the role of community health centers in the U.S.?

4. Which industry trend will have the greatest impact on ambulatory practices? Why?

5. The growth of the ambulatory sector in the U.S. is significant; if you were an entrepreneur, what product or service might you consider for the ambulatory sector? Explain your selection.

REFERENCES

Ambulatory Surgery Center Association. (n.d.). *History.* https://www.ascassociation.org/aboutus/whatisanasc/history#

American Medical Association. (2021). *Physician practice 2020 benchmark survey.*

American Medical Group Association. (n.d.). *AMGA history.* https://www.amga.org/about-amga/amga-difference/amga-history/

Berkowitz, E. (2005). Medicare and Medicaid: The past as prologue. *Health Care Financing Review, 27*(2), 11–23.

Berliner, H. S. (1975). A larger perspective on the Flexner report. *International Journal of Health Services, 5*(4), 573–592. https://doi.org/10.2190/F31Q-592N-056K-VETL

Brook, R. H., Ware, J. E., Rogers, W. H., Keeler, E. B., Davies, A. R., Sherbourne, C. D., & Newhouse, J. P. (1984). *The effect of coinsurance on the health of adults. Results from the RAND health insurance experiment* (R-3055-HHS). RAND Corporation.

Carroll, M. S. (1978). Private health insurance plans in 1976: An evaluation. *Social Security Bulletin, 41*(9), 3–16.

Centers for Disease Control and Prevention. (1999). Achievements in public health, 1900–1999: Changes in the public health system. *Morbidity and Mortality Weekly Report, 48*(50), 1141–1147.

Centers for Disease Control and Prevention. (n.d.). *Outpatient and ambulatory care settings.* https://www.cdc.gov/vhf/ebola/clinicians/outpatient-settings/index.html

Centers for Medicare and Medicaid Services. (2020). *NHE summary, including share of GDP, CY 1960–2019.* U.S. Department of Health and Human Services. https://www.cms.gov/Research-Statistics-Data-and-Systems/Statistics-Trends-and-Reports/NationalHealthExpendData/NationalHealthAccountsHistorical

Cohen, R. A., Makuc, D. M., Bernstein, A. B., Bilheimer, L. T., & Powell-Griner, E. (2009). *Health insurance coverage trends, 1959–2007: Estimates from the National Health Interview Survey* (National Health Statistics Reports No. 17). National Center for Health Statistics.

Collins, S. R., & Aboulafia, G. N. (2021, March 22). Will the American rescue plan reduce the number of uninsured Americans? *To the Point.* Commonwealth Fund. https://doi.org/10.26099/phf6-tn16

Crowley, L. G., & Riordan, C. J. (1988, March/April). Introduction (to conference on medical education in the ambulatory setting). *Journal of General Internal Medicine, 3*(Suppl.), S2–S4.

Davis, M. M. (1927). *Clinics, hospitals and health centers.* Harper & Brothers.

Davis, M. M., & Warner, A. R. (1918). *Dispensaries: Their management and development.* Macmillan.

Deitrick, J. (1966). Most OPD's designed for convenience of administration. *Hospital Topics, 44*(1), 65.

Department of Justice and Federal Trade Commission. (1996, August). *Statements of antitrust enforcement policy in health care.* https://www.justice.gov/atr/page/file/1197731/download

Dudley, R. A., & Luft, H. (2001). Managed care in transition. *New England Journal of Medicine, 344,* 1087–1092. https://doi.org/10.1056/NEJM200104053441410

Ehlke, D. C. (2018). From dispensaries to community health centers: Health delivery change across the twentieth century. *Journal of Community Health, 43,* 625–627. https://doi.org/10.1007/s10900-018-0471-7

Frakes, J. T. (2002, April). Outpatient endoscopy. The case for the ambulatory surgery center. *Gastrointestinal Endoscopy Clinics of North America, 12*(2), 215–227. https://doi.org/10.1016/s1052-5157(01)00004-6

Freeland, M. S., & Schendler, C. E. (1983). National health expenditure growth in the 1980's: An aging population, new technologies, and increasing competition. *Health Care Financing Review, 4*(3), 1–58.

Fye, B. (2016, June 14). The origins and evolution of the mayo clinic. Q&A with Author/Lecturer Bruce Fye, MD. *Circulating Now.* U.S. National Library of Medicine. https://circulatingnow.nlm.nih.gov/2016/06/14/the-origins-and-evolution-of-the-mayo-clinic/

Goldfield, N. (2017, July/September). Dramatic changes in health care professions in the past 40 years. *Journal of Ambulatory Care Management, 40*(3), 169–175. https://doi.org/10.1097/JAC.0000000000000201

Heisler, E. (2018, April 26). *The national health service corps.* Congressional Research Service 7-5700. https://fas.org/sgp/crs/misc/R44970.pdf

Hsiao, W. C., Dunn, D. L., & Verrilli, D. K. (1993). Assessing the implementation of physician payment reform. *New England Journal of Medicine, 328*(13), 928–933. https://doi.org/10.1056/NEJM199304013281306

Institute of Medicine Committee for the Study for the Future of Public Health. (1988). *The future of public health*. National Academies Press.

Institute of Medicine Committee on Quality of Health Care in America. (2001). *Crossing the quality chasm: A new health system for the 21st century*. National Academies Press

Institute of Medicine Committee on the Consequences of Uninsurance. (2002). *Care without coverage: Too little, too late*. National Academies Press. https://www.ncbi.nlm.nih.gov/books/NBK220636/

Keane, C., Marx, J., & Ricci, E. (2001). Privatization and the scope of public health: A national survey of local health department directors. *American Journal of Public Health, 91*(4), 611–617. https://doi.org/10.2105/AJPH.91.4.611

Mayes, R. (2007). The origins, development, and passage of Medicare's revolutionary prospective payment system. *Journal of the History of Medicine and Allied Sciences, 62*(1), 21–55. https://doi.org/10.1093/jhmas/jrj038

Medical Group Management Association. (2021). *Body of knowledge*. https://www.mgma.com/certification/body-of-knowledge

Medical Payment Advisory Commission. (2020, July). *Section 7: Ambulatory care. A data book: Health care spending and the Medicare program*.

Mueller, M. S. (1972). Private health insurance in 1970: Population coverage, enrollment, and financial experience. *Social Security Bulletin, 35*(2), 3–19.

Muhlestein, D., Saunders, R. S., Richards, R., & McClellan, M. B. (2018). Recent progress in the value journey: Growth of ACOs and value-based payment models in 2018. *Health Affairs Blog*, August 14.

Murnaghan, J. H. (1973). Introduction. Supplement: Ambulatory medical care data: Report of the conference on ambulatory medical care records. *Medical Care, 11*(2), 1–5.

National Academies of Medicine. (2021). *Roundtable on population health improvement*. https://www.nationalacademies.org/our-work/roundtable-on-population-health-improvement

National Association of Community Health Centers. (2021, January). *Community health center chartbook*.

Oberlander, J. (2003). *The political life of medicare*. University of Chicago Press.

O'Donnell, B., & Bloniarz, K. (2018, October 4). Medicare payment policies for advanced practice registered nurses (APRNs) and physician assistants (PAs). *MedPAC*. http://www.medpac.gov/docs/default-source/default-document-library/aprn-pa-slide-deck-final-public.pdf?sfvrsn=0

Organisation for Economic Co-operation and Development. (2020). *OECD health statistics 2020*. https://www.oecd.org/health/health-data.htm

Porter, M. E., & Teisberg, E. O. (2006). *Redefining health care: Creating value-based competition on results*. Harvard Business School Press.

Reed, L. (1965). Private health insurance in the United States: An overview. *Bulletin: Social Security, 28*(12), 3–21, 46.

Reed, L., & Hanft, R. (1966, January). National health expenditures, 1950–64. *Bulletin: Social Security, 29*(1), 3–19.

Regenstreif, D. (1977). Innovation in hospital based ambulatory care: Some sources, patterns, and implications of change. *Human Organization, 36*(1), 43–49. https://doi.org/10.17730/humo.36.1.1405786g6g506451

Robinson, J. C. (2001). The end of managed care. *JAMA, 285*(20), 2622–2628. https://doi.org/10.1001/jama.285.20.2622

Roemer, M. (1971). Organized ambulatory health service in international perspective. *International Journal of Health Services, 1*(1), 18–27.

Roemer, M. (1981). Social pressures, not legislation, prompt ambulatory services' growth. *Hospital Progress, 62*(10), 34–39.

Roos, N. P., & Freeman, J. L. (1989). Potential for inpatient-outpatient substitution with diagnosis-related groups. *Health Care Financing Review, 10*(4), 31–38.

Rosenkrantz, B. G. (1972). *Public health and the state: Changing views in Massachusetts, 1842–1936*. Harvard University Press.

Sand, R. (1952). *The advance to social medicine*. Staples Press.

Sia, C., Tonniges, T. F., Osterhus, E., & Taba, S. (2004, May). History of the medical home concept. *Pediatrics, 113*(5, Suppl.), 1473–1478. https://doi.org/10.1542/peds.113.5.S1.1473

Social Security Administration. (n.d.). *History of SSA during the Johnson administration 1963–1968*. https://www.ssa.gov/history/ssa/lbjmedicare1.html

Stoeckle, J. D., Stoeckle, A. L., Grossman, J. H., & Goroll, A. H. (1979). A case history of training outside the hospital and its future. *The American Journal of Medicine, 66*(6), 1008–1014. https://doi.org/10.1016/0002-9343(79)90458-3

Taylor, J. (2004). *The fundamentals of community health centers* (NHPF Background Paper). National Health Policy Forum, George Washington University http://lib.ncfh.org/pdfs/2k9/8142.pdf

Tolbert, J., Kendal Orgera, K., & Damico, A. (2020, November). *Key facts about the uninsured population*. Kaiser Family Foundation. https://www.kff.org/uninsured/issue-brief/key-facts-about-the-uninsured-population/

United States Bureau of Labor Statistics. (2020, September 1). *Table 2.7: Employment and output by industry*. https://www.bls.gov/emp/tables/industry-employment-and-output.htm

University of Michigan School of Public Health. (1968). *Medical care chart book*. Bureau of Public Health Economics.

STRATEGY AND LEADERSHIP

WITH CONTRIBUTING AUTHOR JALANA MCCASLAND

LEARNING OBJECTIVES

1. Explain the importance of strategic planning in ambulatory practices
2. Describe the elements of **strategic intent**
3. Articulate the steps of the strategic planning process
4. Depict the role of leadership and management in the realization of identified strategies

KEY TERMS

Competition	Strategic Plan
Strategic Intent	Environmental Analysis
Stakeholders	Strategic Alternatives
Core Competency	Psychological Safety

INTRODUCTION

Strategy development and execution are essential to every organization. Providing a road map for the organization, a **strategic plan** translates the values, vision, and mission of an organization into action. For organizations to succeed, they must interpret the current landscape and trends, craft and communicate a cogent strategic intent, assess and develop the capacity for change, forge and execute plans with conviction, and continually learn from their actions. For the well-managed ambulatory practice, the creation and implementation of a strategic plan provide essential guidance to successfully navigate the impact of internal and external forces. As the environment for an ambulatory practice is ever-changing, strategy development requires both leadership vision and attention to detail. Because strategic planning is essential to long-term viability, every ambulatory practice can and should engage in it, regardless of the practice's size or organizational structure.

STRATEGY

The ambulatory environment demands attention to strategy as **competition** is fierce, technology is rapidly evolving, and patients demand not only quality care but convenient access and exceptional service as well. A well-managed ambulatory practice understands these challenges and seeks to proactively address them instead of simply reacting to them.

Although a singular term, a *strategy*—and the planning process to articulate one—is a continuous, iterative process rather than a distinct event. The planning cycle begins with visioning and setting goals, developing objectives and tactics to achieve that vision, monitoring performance, adjusting as needed based on business intelligence, and continuously reflecting and revising the plan. Historically, ambulatory practices used a horizon of 10 years into the future for strategic planning. However, given the uncertainty of today's healthcare environment, the horizon is typically one to three years. Strategic planning is not a final destination but rather an ongoing journey that must be constantly revisited.

Roles and Responsibilities

Developing a strategy is a continuous process of assessment, learning, and adjustment. Strategy—and the plans that emanate from the development of one—requires a thoughtful approach. The ambulatory practice must create a formal structure for strategic planning, establish or update the organization's strategic intent, and take steps to develop the plan. Developing successful strategies requires the active participation of everyone in the ambulatory practice; however, key **stakeholders** play an important role in the coordination and oversight for the development and execution of the strategic plan. The roles and responsibilities for strategy development include the governing body and the practice's leaders and managers. The stakeholders incorporate physicians and other clinical leaders, as well as the administrator(s) of the practice.

Governing Body

The composition of a governing board varies across ambulatory organizations. For many ambulatory practices, the governing body is comprised of the managing partners, who are typically physicians. The administrator may also be a member of the board. The governing body leads the practice's effort in strategy development and planning. Smaller physician practices may be owned and operated by a physician owner or founder who sets the direction for a strategic plan, with input from others within the practice and perhaps with the support of a third-party consultant or advisor. Some ambulatory practices may not have a true governing board but rather an executive group composed of key physician leaders who execute strategy.

Ambulatory practices owned or operated by a hospital or health system typically fall under the auspices of the facility's board of trustees. The board of trustees resides at the corporate level and is responsible for coordinating the development and approval of the health system's strategic plan. The systemwide plan may include a component focused on the ambulatory enterprise, just as it would for inpatient, skilled nursing, and the other service lines of the health system. For the ambulatory component, the strategic planning process is often delegated to physicians and administrative leaders with ambulatory expertise. They are selected to craft a strategy for the ambulatory enterprise that aligns with the health system's goals.

Regardless of composition, the governing body plays three important roles in the strategy development process: surveillance, capacity building, and stakeholder identification and engagement.

Surveillance

The governing board sets the overall direction of an organization by establishing its values, vision, and mission. The formation of these strategic intents may only occur once in the history of the organization; however, they may be updated particularly if there is a major change to the organization, such as a merger or an acquisition. On an ongoing basis, the governing board serves a surveillance role. In this position, the board not only identifies and acknowledges opportunities but also serves to challenge assumptions (Orlikoff & Totten, 2006). Governing boards must balance the need to be good stewards of the organization while at the same time making crucial decisions for future investments (Orlikoff & Totten, 2006). This corporate-level perspective is important in setting the tone and direction for the strategic plan.

Capacity Building

Another role the governing body plays in the strategy development and planning process relates to capacity building. The continual assessment of the organization's capabilities and competencies provides insight into the ability of the organization to achieve its desired results. For example, if the ambulatory practice's strategy is to shift the care delivery model to place greater emphasis on prevention and wellness—a population health management strategy—the governing body would need to assess the current capabilities and competencies within the practice to effectively execute the strategy. A successful strategic plan is not only one that inspires and motivates action but one that is also practical and achievable. If the strategic plan needs resources or technology, the governing body must prioritize integrating those resources, or capacity building, within the other needs of the ambulatory practice.

Stakeholder Identification and Engagement

The third role of the governing body as it relates to strategy development and planning is identifying and engaging relevant stakeholders. Relevant stakeholders are those committed to the organization's strategic intent and in a position to influence the attainment of the desired results. The board ensures stakeholder input is incorporated into the strategic planning process and that stakeholders' needs and expectations drive the organization's goals. For example, in crafting an ambulatory strategy for a hospital, physician participation in the strategic planning process at the board level as a key stakeholder is essential. The board may also solicit input from key community leaders or other partners or affiliates who can provide an additional external perspective on what the community or region needs. This input is essential in crafting a strategic plan that not only meets the needs of the key practice stakeholders (providers, staff, and patients) but also delivers value to the community.

Ambulatory Practice Leaders

The input of physicians and other clinicians serving in the practice is key in the development and execution of the strategic plan. Clinical leaders often serve as change leaders or champions to help operationalize the plan. Similarly, ambulatory leaders such as the practice administrator or manager and other key clinical and administrative leaders provide important input as well as help assess the practice's capacity and willingness to adopt the strategic plan.

Larger ambulatory practices or those embedded within hospitals or health systems may have a senior official, such as a vice president or a director of strategy, who manages the strategic planning process. Practices may also engage the services of a third-party consultant to assist with certain aspects of the strategic planning process, specifically as it relates to moderating the planning session; offer intelligence regarding industry trends; or solicit and report on insight gleaned from patients or referral sources. A third party may also be in the best position to interview the practice's personnel and present blinded findings regarding themes and opportunities for improvement.

Every ambulatory practice can engage in strategic planning. However, the strategic planning process is additive to the work of the physicians and leaders who are already busy overseeing daily operations. While the roles and responsibilities may vary depending on the size of the practice and can often be shared between members, the time needed to devote to a strategic planning process should not be underestimated. For this reason, the practice must clearly articulate the roles and responsibilities of the individuals engaged in the strategic planning process. Doing so avoids duplication and makes the best use of the practice's resources.

Strategic Intent

Strategic intent is an organization's overarching purpose; it is crucial to determine the alignment of strategy with the mission, vision, and values of the organization. The purpose serves to inform stakeholders of the organization's commitment to its direction and functions as a basis upon which to measure success. As an otolaryngology practice, should we open an ambulatory surgery center? As a multispecialty practice, should we launch a transitional care management clinic? As an ambulatory enterprise of a health system, should we invest in a nurse contact center? What purpose will these strategies serve? Do they align with the practice's values, mission, and vision? These are questions that can best be addressed by understanding strategic intent. Strategies, like enzymes, are catalysts, which lead to a desired outcome or change. Strategies guide behaviors, which, in turn, are used to steer actions and subsequently achieve results.

In *The Theory of Business*, Peter Drucker suggests that an organization's failure to thrive is not based on doing the wrong things or doing things wrong; rather, he states, failure is related to the "assumptions on which the organization has been built and is being run no longer fit reality" (Drucker, 1994, p. 95). These assumptions, he asserts, "shape an organization's behavior, dictate its decisions about what to do and what not to do, and define what the organization considers meaningful results" (Drucker, 1994, p. 96). Understanding an organization's strategic intent is a fundamental first step in the strategy process.

Values, vision, and mission are the elements that contribute to defining strategic intent (see Figure 2.1). Values are the shared concepts and beliefs the ambulatory practice and its members hold dear; they are the core principles that guide behavior. The vision is a future-oriented statement of the practice's purpose and how the practice wants others to view it. The vision is aspirational and identifies where the organization wants to be in the future. The mission is used to communicate an organization's business today. A mission statement captures the practice's reason for being and reflects the present.

Strategic Plan

Strategy is the catalyst that makes possible the achievement of desired outcomes, serving to guide behaviors and achieve organizational vision and mission, all while being true to the organizational values. A strategic plan is the result of creating and documenting the organization's strategies. Using the analogy of constructing a building, the organization's strategic intent (values, vision, and mission) serves as the building's blueprint, a guide to the organization's desired results (see Figure 2.2). The strategic plan, a conglomeration of individual strategies designed to achieve the purpose of the organization, supports the building's foundation. Each strategy is then organized

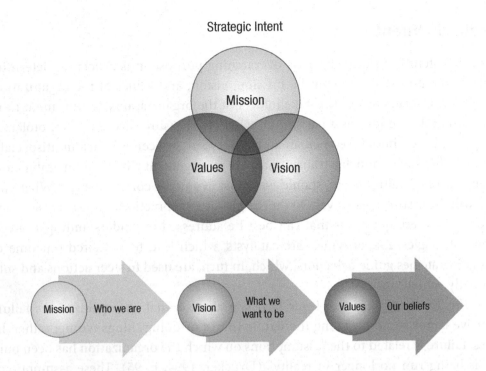

FIGURE 2.1 Strategic intent.

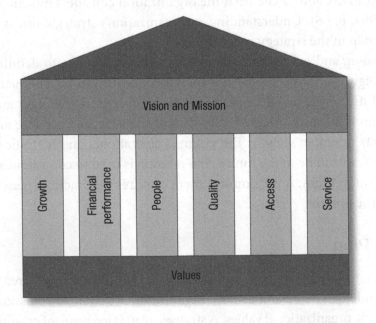

FIGURE 2.2 Strategic pillars.

and the execution coordinated; this provides a framework for action, much like the studs and joists used to frame a building. The alignment of coordinated strategies is referred to as the organization's strategic plan.

The process of strategic planning allows a practice to maintain one eye on the future—leading—and the other eye on the present—managing—with a purpose and conviction reflective of the organization's values, vision, and mission.

For many ambulatory practices, an effective way to organize this work is to establish pillars based on the organization's strategic intent. For example, recruiting and retaining personnel who support the values, mission, and vision of an ambulatory practice is essential to its success. By creating a "people" pillar, the practice recognizes the importance of its human capital. The strategic plan may include an objective to attract and retain top-performing personnel to the organization. The tactic determined to meet this goal may be to offer and maintain market-competitive compensation and benefits. Actions that may emanate from the tactic are a biannual market compensation review, an employee engagement survey, the formation of a compensation task force, and an analysis of exit interviews from prior periods.

An effective visual cue for stakeholders involved in the strategic planning process—as well as those engaged in it as personnel of the practice—the pillars connect the organization's mission and vision to its stated values. Pillars are unique to each practice and should be derived from the organization's values. Pillars for consideration in an ambulatory practice include people, access, quality, financial performance, growth, and service. The number of pillars should be reasonable; easily communicated to the practice providers, staff, and other stakeholders; and reflective of the practice's strategic intent.

STEPS TO DEVELOP A STRATEGIC PLAN

The steps to develop a strategic plan, as outlined in Figure 2.3, include conducting the **environmental analysis**, developing **strategic alternatives**, creating strategic goals and objectives, creating an action plan, executing the plan, and evaluating progress toward the desired goals. Strategic planning is an iterative process as each strategy is evaluated and adjustments made based on performance or changes to the underlying assumptions based on new data.

Step 1: Conduct an Environmental Analysis

The environmental analysis is an assessment of an organization's internal capabilities and competencies as well as a reflection on the external landscape. An environmental analysis is not a matter of conjecture or opinion or based solely on subjective input from key stakeholders. While important, stakeholder input is just one component of data collection. Factual data and business intelligence about the internal and external environment provide the foundation for the analysis. A well-managed ambulatory practice relies on an evidence-informed planning process. Using objective tools, appropriately and for the intended purpose, reduces biases, encourages broad-based

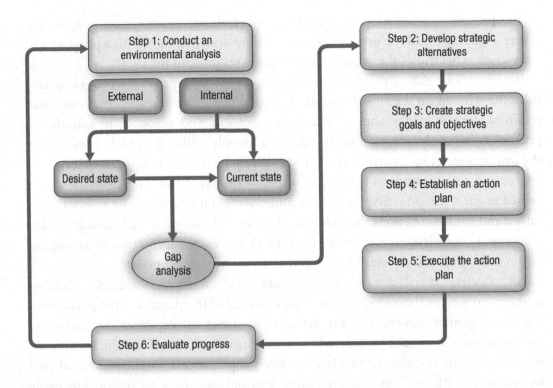

FIGURE 2.3 The steps to developing a strategic plan.

SOURCE: Adapted from Walston, S. L. (2013). *Strategic healthcare management: Planning and execution.* Health Administration Press

participation in the data gathering and analysis process, and provides a platform on which to inform the creation of strategic options and decision-making. The data gathered through the environmental analysis create the underlying assumptions that drive the success of the planning process.

The environmental analysis is not a onetime process. Rather, organizations should develop a process for continual surveillance, interpretation, discussion, and the sharing of relevant findings on an ongoing basis. The data and information garnered from these analyses, both internal and external, are used to inform the development of new strategies as well as assess progress and identify opportunities in existing strategies.

Internal Analysis

The internal analysis is concerned with understanding the alignment of the strategic intent with organizational capabilities and competencies. *Organizational capability* is a broad term that defines the organization's capacity to "deploy resources that have been purposefully integrated to achieve the desired end state" and represent "the collective skills, abilities, and expertise of an organization" (Ulrich & Smallwood, 2004).

Capabilities, to include the ability to adapt or execute efficiently, are key intangible assets. According to Dave Ulrich and Norm Smallwood (2004), "you can't see or touch [capabilities], yet they can make all the difference in the world when it comes to market value, and are the outcome of investments in staffing, training, compensation, communication, and other human resources areas" (Ulrich & Smallwood, 2004, p. 119).

Organizational competencies refer to the ability of an organization to achieve its purpose. Prahalad and Hamel (1990) coined the term *core competence* to distinguish those capabilities fundamental to an organization's performance and strategy—and those that provide it with a competitive advantage. Using the analogy of tree roots designed to give and propel growth, **core competencies** are "the collective learning in the organization," according to Prahalad and Hamel (1990, p. 81).

Conducting an internal analysis, the well-managed ambulatory practice seeks to understand current capabilities and competencies as well as consider what may be needed in the future. The internal analysis incorporates resource availability, allocation, and use. Resources include people, facilities, technology, equipment, and finances.

Data collected from the internal assessment after analysis and validation are used for an internal gap analysis. The internal gap analysis answers questions about the current and future state: Where are we now, and where do we need to be to achieve our chosen results? As gaps are identified, the organization must be prepared to reallocate existing resources or invest in new resources to close the identified gaps. For example, if the practice's desire to develop a population health management strategy includes the creation of a nurse contact center focused on ambulatory health promotion and the internal assessment reveals there is no capability or competencies within the organization related to this new venture, a gap has been identified. The gap in capability and competencies can be filled through the hiring of new talent (i.e., a senior nurse leader with contact center experience), developing talents in existing personnel (i.e., recruiting nurses from other areas in the practice and training them in ambulatory health promotion), or accessing sought-after skills through alliances or partnerships with people (i.e., a population health consultant) or organizations possessing the requisite competencies (i.e., create a joint venture with an existing nurse contact center). Considerations will also need to be given to additional gaps identified: How will data be collected and reported? Is additional technology needed to support the contact center? These gaps in people, facilities, technology, equipment, and finances will need to be identified and addressed for the plan to be successful.

Questions to consider related to the internal analysis include the following:

1. How does the organization bundle resources to build capabilities and core competencies that create value?
2. Could the organization align its resources in a better way to improve its capabilities and core competencies?

3. Is it likely that environmental changes will make the organization's capabilities and core competencies obsolete?

4. Are substitutes for the organization's capabilities and core competencies available or soon to be available?

5. Could the organization's capabilities and core competencies easily be imitated?

6. How can the organization best protect or improve its capabilities and core competencies?

Leaders should continually assess and invest in building capabilities and core competencies in areas aligned with the organization's strategic intent.

Ambulatory practices should also be familiar with their internal data and historical trends. For example, is the volume of patients increasing or decreasing? Is the number of new patients growing as a percent of total encounters? What services are those new patients seeking? From which sources are referrals to the practice coming? Are certain referral sources increasing or decreasing the number of referrals to the practice? Are we able to schedule the referrals, or are we losing referrals? Comparing key practice data—by month, quarter, or year—may highlight areas of opportunity; Table 2.1 offers a list of elements that an ambulatory practice may evaluate to gain insight—and data that may offer a better understanding of the area of interest. This list is not exhaustive; every ambulatory practice should consider key data elements that can be tracked year over year and are meaningful to its strategic planning process.

External Analysis

The external analysis is focused on gathering intelligence on a host of factors related to the environment outside of the practice, including the competitive, regulatory, political, technological, and financial landscape.

There are several tools and techniques for completing an external assessment. These tools, which may also incorporate the internal analysis, include stakeholder analysis, SWOT (strengths, weaknesses, opportunities, and threats) analysis, PEST (political, economic, social, and technology) analysis, scenario analysis, financial analysis, portfolio analysis, and value-chain analysis (Walston, 2013, pp. 181–208). Each of these tools can prove valuable to an ambulatory practice; Figure 2.4 displays a sample PEST analysis for an ambulatory practice. These reliable strategic planning tools provide credible frameworks for the collection and analysis of both quantitative and qualitative data.

Hospitals report inpatient admission data, which are publicly available and easily accessible; however, obtaining market-based ambulatory data can be difficult. Claims data are available for Medicare outpatient services; other data may be purchased from third parties. However, the data may not be comprehensive or reflective of the ambulatory practice (particularly for a single-specialty practice), thus making

TABLE 2.1 Elements for Evaluation in an Ambulatory Practice

INSIGHT	DATA
TALENT	Average lead time to recruit by position; employee attrition rate by position; the average tenure of employees (those who stay and those who leave); employee engagement survey; exit interviews
DEMAND	Inbound referrals by specialty: referral sources, volume, turnaround time, and leakage; CPT® codes: volume and frequency; communication volume by mode (calls, chats, texts, messages)
PRODUCTIVITY	Encounters; work-relative value units, charges by clinician; clinic sessions worked per year as compared to expected/contracted
CAPACITY	Total number of visits compared to industry standards by specialty; volume of unused appointment slots; slot utilization; appointment no-show and last-minute cancelation rate; clinician bump rate
ACUITY	Diagnosis codes; volume and frequency; evaluation and management code levels
MARKET	Payer mix by site; percentage of physicians in the community by specialty; appointment lag time for new patients by specialty
QUALITY	Patient-reported outcome measures; National Quality Forum measures (process, cost/resource use, outcome, structure); payer performance related to quality measures
GROWTH	Encounters; new patient encounters as a percentage of total encounters; volume of new-to-practice patients ("net new")
PATIENT SATISFACTION	Net Promoter Score; Clinician and Group Consumer Assessment of Healthcare Providers and Systems survey results over time; search engine ratings for practice or provider

Political

Telemedicine regulations uncertain

Physician referral law

Medicaid expansion at the state level

Stable local governement

Provider-friendly insurance commissioner elected for coming term; may combat trends in slow payments; denials

Economic

Growing unemployment in community leading to rising uninsured rates

Largest employer closing in short term (~1 year); potential shift in payer mix

Economic growth in adjacent markets, but primary markets in decline

Low inflation rates

Shortage in labor markets for medical assistants

Social

Heightened patient expectations for sevice, access, and convenience

High bad debt

Average age of community increasing (~55 YOA); pediatric population decreasing

Growing need for mental health

Technology

Opportunity to expand virtual care offerings

Expanding access to social determinants of health data

Integration of artificial intelligence in administrative processes

FIGURE 2.4 Sample ambulatory practice PEST analysis.

it directional at best. How then can the ambulatory practice obtain reliable and valid data on the external environment?

One way to conduct an environmental analysis is to identify and evaluate market trends that impact or influence the ambulatory practice. For example, an obstetrics and gynecology practice may review birth rates in its local market. Are the number of births in the area decreasing, flat, or increasing? These data are accessible, and when reviewed in conjunction with trends in practice volume, the collective data may signal an increase or decrease in practice market share.

Ambulatory practices can stay abreast of external trends is by joining and participating in professional associations. Meetings of state medical associations, national special societies, local coalitions of practice managers, or other groups may highlight trends that may impact the operations of the practice and offer networking opportunities that allow intelligence to be shared among members. Finally, the ambulatory practice administrator can run a simple keyword search on "trends in ambulatory care." The search can be customized to a specific date range, providing the most relevant news and articles to the strategic planning period.

As previously discussed, obtaining stakeholder input is essential. Reviewing patient or referring physician satisfaction survey data or organizing focus groups with select patients or key referral sources are ways to collect these data. If conducting a focus group, consider using a trained facilitator who can help guide the discussion and summarize the key takeaways.

Similar to the internal analysis, the results of the external analysis provide the basis for comparison between the current state and the desired state. Where gaps are identified, the organization must be committed to closing the identified gaps.

Step 2: Develop Strategic Alternatives

Once the environmental analysis is complete, it is time to consider the strategic alternatives. To this point, we have treated the environmental analysis as a singular event, when, in fact, it is an iterative process. Once the strategic plan is in place, regularly reassessing the environment and looking for gaps is part of the cyclical nature of the strategic planning process.

Let's consider an example related to the growth of an orthopedic practice. Our external analysis has revealed that the local government is building a new recreational center to attract local, regional, and national sports teams as part of its tourism strategy. The practice treats sports injuries but does not have a physician, advanced practice provider, or personnel specifically trained in sports medicine. How should the orthopedic practice respond?

■ **Work with local government officials to determine opportunities.** What investments would the community be willing to make to support this aspect of their tourism strategy? Does the governing board have an existing relationship with community leaders that can offer insight into specific community needs and expectations? What are the expectations of the local government as it relates to healthcare for the new recreational center? Will it be choosing a preferred medical provider for the facility, or will the teams be selecting their own?

- **Build the internal capability to meet this potential new demand.** Does the practice have providers interested in sports medicine? If not, should the practice acquire this expertise either through recruitment or additional training by existing personnel? Are there providers in the market who could be recruited to fulfill this need? Should the practice invest in personnel such as athletic trainers or ancillaries related to the service such as mobile imaging? Are these services reimbursed? How many personnel would need to be recruited or acquired to be effective? What is the return on investment? What other capability should the practice develop to engage with the recreational center?

- **Develop affiliation or partnership agreements with other providers to offer the full continuum of services.** Should the practice partner with an external provider or facility to offer medical, training, therapy, imaging, and/or rehabilitation services? Are there alternative relationships that may serve the purpose of fulfilling this opportunity?

- **Merge with another practice that already has existing sports medicine expertise.** Does the practice have the interest but lack the capacity or resources to meet this new demand? Could a merger with another practice fulfill this opportunity—and perhaps others? How would the merged practices collaborate to meet this need? What identified gaps can merging the two practices resolve? How would the merged practices complement one another to address specific needs such as same-day access, weekend, evening, and emergent hours? Could there be a greater benefit (than simply the recreational center) for a merger?

- **Do nothing.** If the practice does not react, what, if any, is the expected response from competitors regarding the opportunity? Will the recreational center pursue opportunities outside of the local market if the needs are not fulfilled by the practice or a competitor in the market? If so, what are the implications of these activities?

There may be additional options for the practice to consider. Each of the possible strategic alternatives needs to be evaluated thoroughly. The alternatives should also be assessed against the organization's strategic intent. Which alternative allows the practice to fulfill its mission and vision? Does the chosen strategic alternative align with its values? Each alternative should be vetted by key stakeholders to ensure their views and opinions are heard. The alternatives should also be considered in light of regulatory, financial, and resource requirements. How will this impact other projects? Do we have the time and resources to pursue this option given other opportunities being considered? Can we afford not to pursue this opportunity? What changes should be considered in the existing strategic plan to take advantage of this potential new strategy? Finally, the competitive landscape is crucial to examine; if we decide not to pursue the opportunity, who will? What are the implications of a competitor engaging with the recreation center opportunity?

Once the strategic alternative is selected, the next step is to create the goals and objectives that will be used to guide execution.

Step 3: Create Strategic Goals and Objectives

In this phase of the planning process, the strategic alternative has been selected. Let us assume that the decision is made to merge with another orthopedic practice to build the resources and capacity to meet this potential new demand, take advantage of other opportunities related to growth in the orthopedic market, and prevent competitors from entering the market. The governing bodies of both practices, in this example, may become the managing physician partners of the newly merged practice. The managing partners direct the practice administrator from each practice to form a planning committee, composed of key providers and personnel, to develop a merger plan. Within this complex process, for simplicity in this example, the groups elect to focus on the following key areas through a phased approach: creating an organizational hierarchy, integrating staff payroll and benefit plans, and establishing a unified set of policies and procedures. For each area of focus, goals, and objectives need to be determined. The goals and objectives should follow the SMART principles for goal setting: specific, measurable, attainable, relevant, and time-bound.

Step 4: Establish an Action Plan

The action plan consists of specific tasks that must be accomplished to achieve the objectives. Furthermore, it is critical to establish accountability by identifying the persons who will be held responsible for executing each task. A project plan can facilitate the documentation of the progress steps, accountable individual(s), time frame, and assessment metric(s) for each task. Considering the execution of each task is essential.

For the orthopedic practice engaged in the merger as an example, communication regarding the organizational change is essential, but the timing of the announcement must be considered. The practice does not want to communicate too soon to prompt a competitive response from another individual or organization; however, neither does the practice want to risk the ill will of providers, staff, patients, and stakeholders by communicating too late. In sum, communication must be managed. Therefore, an

BOX 2.1	RECOMMENDATIONS FOR THE EXECUTION OF A STRATEGIC PLAN

1. Keep it simple, and make it concrete
2. Debate assumptions, not forecasts
3. Use a rigorous framework, and speak a common language
4. Discuss resource deployments early
5. Concisely identify priorities
6. Continuously monitor performance
7. Reward and develop execution capabilities

SOURCE: Adapted from Mankins, M., & Steele, R. (2005, July/August). Turning great strategy into great performance. *Harvard Business Review, 83*(7/8), 64–72.

action item would be "develop a thoughtful, appropriate communication plan that provides key messaging to providers, staff, patients, and stakeholders." Within the action plan will be milestones that need to be achieved, accompanied by when and who is responsible for ensuring the completion. Performance metrics will also be implemented to measure success.

Step 5: Execute the Action Plan

A strategy is guaranteed to fail without effective execution. Is it better to have a lackluster strategy that is expertly executed, or a thoughtful strategy that is executed poorly? Not having a clearly articulated, evidence-informed strategy places organizations at significant risk. However, having a deliberate, relevant strategy is also no guarantee of success. Effective execution is essential. Organizations typically realize only a portion of their strategies' potential value because of breakdowns in planning and implementation. The strategy-to-performance gap was recognized by management experts Mankins and Steele (2005), who offered recommendations in Box 2.1 to enhance the likelihood of the successful execution of a strategic plan.

Among organizations with a clearly defined strategy, many do not produce the desired change. These failures are in part due to missteps in execution. There are other factors associated with this performance, including challenges related to leadership, communication, decision-making, accountability, and an understanding of the organization's readiness and capacity for change.

Successful strategic planning requires deliberate oversight by the governing body and accountability by the leaders responsible for development and implementation. Without a plan or accountability for results, actions may be misdirected or lack the precision and focus needed for successful execution.

Step 6: Evaluate Progress

Once the strategic plan's execution is underway, the planning cycle reverts to the reflection phase. This step, which is better considered an iterative process, involves collecting data on performance, monitoring progress along the charted course, and making adjustments as needed to keep the practice heading toward the ultimate desired outcome. Practices use a variety of instruments to monitor performance. Some practices use a RASCI (responsible, accountable, support, consulted, and informed) tool to assign a responsible party to a specific objective. Other practices may create a dashboard or a balanced scorecard that measures the completion of strategic objectives using a visual cue such as red, yellow, and green coloring to denote progress. A performance monitoring instrument provides a framework for managing the implementation of strategy, focusing attention on the importance of the strategy by all stakeholders.

Whichever tool is chosen, it should be simple to use, easy to understand, and provide a status summary that can be shared with practice providers, staff, and stakeholders at regular intervals.

Achieving the desired objectives and tactics is essential to a successful plan. Equally important, however, is a plan that can be modified and adapted due to a change in the internal or external environment. This is where feedback and learning become important. The data collected may be used to make adjustments. Stakeholders should be rewarded for the application of evidence as they seek to improve performance. Regular communication using a consistent tool ensures that strategic planning is an ongoing, iterative process rather than a single event.

FUTURES WHEEL

Most ambulatory practices engage in some type of strategic planning, whether it may be planning for a new service line, upgrading new software, or assessing the impact of competition. Plans are formulated to adapt and respond to a change in the internal or external environment. Traditional strategic planning, carefully prepared and monitored, can yield performance improvements. Practices may opt to enhance their strategic planning efforts by engaging in a process called "strategic foresight." The six steps included in strategic foresight include framing, scanning, forecasting, visioning, planning, and acting (Hines & Bishop, 2015). Strategic foresight takes a deeper look at issues or challenges facing the ambulatory practice. The technique provides a framework for the ambulatory practice to develop and choose among several possible future strategic alternatives.

One tool used in strategic foresight is the "futures wheel." Invented in 1972 by Jerome C. Glenn, the futures wheel visually displays primary, secondary, and tertiary

FUTURES WHEEL: INCREASING WELLNESS VISITS

To enhance preventive health for its patient population, an academic family practice division used the futures wheel exercise. The aim was to increase wellness visits to Medicare patients, a key preventive service provided to patients in the division's ambulatory practice. While traditional planning yielded some improvements, the division struggled to meet its budgeted targets for these important preventive maintenance visits. To date, outreach efforts to schedule Medicare patients for wellness visits had been largely met with refusal, cancelation, or no-shows. To gain further insight into how to increase Medicare wellness visits, the division's leadership brought together physicians, nurses, and supervisors, led by a trained facilitator, to brainstorm alternatives using a Futures Wheel. Medicare wellness visits were placed at the center of the wheel as the problem or issue needing attention. Using an expanded PEST Analysis by gathering and assessing the STEEPLE (social, technology, economic, environmental, political, legal, and ethical) criteria, the facilitator led the division's representatives through a brainstorming exercise to identify the primary and secondary impact of each factor on the wellness visits. During the brainstorming session, the practice was encouraged to shout out all ideas or suggestions. For example, while discussing social factors impacting the wellness visits, the group discussed that patients' unfamiliarity with the purpose of the visits led to a secondary impact of appointment no-shows, cancelations, or refusal. Another direct social impact was the provider culture, which generated little support for visits among staff. The practice brainstormed direct and indirect impacts for all of the STEEPLE criteria. The futures wheel (see Figure 2.5) provided a comprehensive view of direct (first-order) and indirect (second-order) factors impacting wellness visits. The futures wheel was then posted in the department so that all providers and staff could continue to brainstorm potential impacts. Subsequent division meetings used the information to develop action plans.

consequences of events, trends, emerging issues, and future potential alternatives (Glenn, 2009). A futures wheel also identifies various strategic alternatives and gives the end-user insight into the impact of choosing one strategic alternative over another (see the sidebar Futures Wheel: Increasing Wellness Visits for an example of using the futures wheel). While traditional strategic planning provides the well-managed ambulatory practice with a specific road map, strategic foresight provides the practice with several potential strategic alternatives. Flexibility and adaptability give the ambulatory practice an even greater opportunity for success in today's fast-paced healthcare industry.

LEADERSHIP

Leadership plays an essential role in the development of the strategic plan and ensuring its success in furthering the practice's strategic intent. Each strategy within a

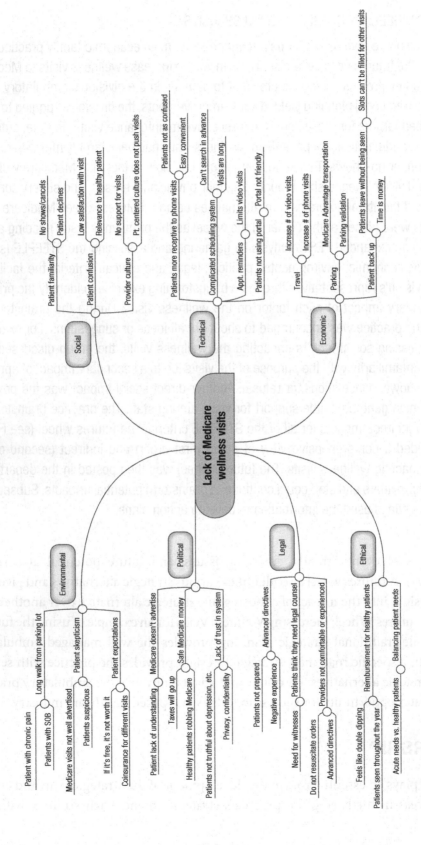

FIGURE 2.5 Futures wheel.

strategic plan provides a framework for action, much like the studs and joists used to frame a building. Leadership is like the roof, holding the building together and making it sustainable. The well-managed ambulatory practice engages leaders at all levels, formal and informal, in the strategic planning process.

Formal leadership roles vary in the ambulatory practice depending on the organization. For example, in large hospital settings, a medical director of ambulatory services may provide executive oversight for the ambulatory enterprise in concert with a vice president of ambulatory services. Together, these individuals form a leadership dyad that may be replicated throughout the ambulatory organization. The primary care service line, for example, may have the same dyad with a medical director and administrator; the leadership model may be duplicated in other service lines such as oncology, musculoskeletal, and cardiac care. In other ambulatory practices, the formal leader may be the physician founder or owner. Alternatively, the governing board may hire a practice administrator who is responsible not only for the strategy of the practice but also for the daily operations.

Roles and Responsibilities

The particulars of the organizational structure are not as important as having a clear understanding of the roles and responsibilities of each member of the leadership team along with a dedication to good communication, respect for each other's expertise, and an understanding and commitment to the organization's strategic intent. One of the most critical jobs of the leadership team is engaging providers and staff who will be implementing the proposed strategy. It is the leader's responsibility to build a process that allows everyone's input to be heard. For example, clinicians engaged in direct patient care bring valuable insight regarding the clinical processes of care delivery and can also represent the voices of their patients. For ambulatory practices, the perspectives of clinicians are especially meaningful given the heterogeneity of the ambulatory sector. In choosing among strategic alternatives, it is also critically important that ambulatory leaders consider the diversity of their patients, staff, and stakeholders. If conducting a patient or employee focus group, ensure the group has representation from the population it serves.

Ambulatory leaders should also create **psychological safety**, which allows for the critical review and evaluation of proposed strategic alternatives. In a psychologically safe environment, people feel comfortable speaking and offering ideas and feedback without being criticized or punished (Edmondson & Lei, 2014). Allowing for honest and candid feedback among strategic alternatives is essential to developing a strategic plan that engages providers and staff. In gathering responses, a leader should not assume silence is agreement. Instead, a process built through a survey or another form of anonymous feedback allows everyone an opportunity to provide input. Some practices may distribute a copy of the draft strategic plan to each provider and staff member, giving them ample time to reflect and comment on the strategy; other practices may post a copy of the strategy on an intranet site or key area in the practice to allow providers and staff to comment. Never underestimate the importance of communicating early and often with the practice's providers and staff.

Once the strategic alternatives are appropriately vetted and the decision to proceed along a given path is made, the leadership team is charged with developing the action plan and tactics along with a timeline for completion. Further, leaders must engage the support of the providers and staff to achieve the desired results.

Strategic Planning Skills

The practice leader may be a physician executive, a practice administrator, or a combination of the two. Regardless of the organizational structure, leading an ambulatory practice is challenging. Ambulatory practice leadership styles are as varied as the organizational structures within which they operate. For this chapter, the focus is on the key skills necessary for the leader during the strategic planning process (see the sidebar The Importance of Emotional Intelligence in Healthcare Leadership for the value of emotional intelligence). As it relates to strategic planning, the critical abilities of ambulatory practice leaders include the following:

1. **Collaboration.** The leader must collaborate with his or her physician colleague as part of the leadership dyad responsible for the strategic planning process. If no formal leadership dyad exists, the leader engages with informal physician leaders. Seek those physician leaders who are willing to provide honest feedback—and those who embrace change as well as representatives who are typically resistant. Engage personnel, as well as physicians. The strategic planning process should challenge the team to question the status quo and to brainstorm future strategic alternatives. Contesting the status quo—"how we have always done things"—may be uncomfortable for some providers and staff. However, if managed appropriately, the process may yield critical insights for strategic plan development and execution.

   Conflict is inevitable as decisions are made regarding strategies, tactics, and actions; it can create negative feelings that may derail the strategic planning process. A collaborative leader refocuses the conflict away from the negative emotions and toward the best interests of the practice and the patients it serves. Research suggests that more diverse teams produce better results (Ibarra & Hansen, 2011). The collaborative leader recognizes the richness found in diversity, acknowledges the uncomfortableness, and leads the team forward by building transparency and trust in the process by being open and receptive to the dialogue.

2. **Teambuilding.** During the strategic planning process, the leader must ensure clarity regarding the roles and responsibilities of each stakeholder. To avoid duplication, team members must be clear on the roles they perform

during the strategic planning process and the responsibilities others conduct (Levi & Askay, 2020). A leader is also responsible for building group cohesion. Fostering group solidarity builds a sense of unity and connects the team members to the practice's strategic intent, as well as its strategic plan. Practices embarking on a strategic planning process should consider the strength of their team structure before the planning process begins and take proactive steps to increase cohesion through team-building activities.

3. **Change Leadership.** Behavior change impedes the implementation of new initiatives. Whether the alteration is something relatively straightforward, such as adding a new screening tool to the arrival process, or something far more complex, like implementing a new billing system, persuading practitioners to adopt new ways to work requires behavior modification. Change is difficult. Leaders use their influence to help others see the value in making the change. Leaders tell the story of why a change is necessary and how it may benefit the practice. Furthermore, leaders help individuals determine the role that they can play in facilitating change.

    Physician leaders can serve as champions among physicians for the desired change. The physician champion serves as an early adopter, acting to role model the desired behaviors. Early adopters lead by example, demonstrating the benefits of the new system and serving as a resource to others as they adopt the new process. Early adopters also help identify and resolve unanticipated issues that may arise with the new process.

4. **Focus.** Leadership, as Peter Drucker said, is about doing the right thing; management is about doing things right (Drucker, 2000). Within an ambulatory practice, the lines between leadership and management are often blurred. Particularly for small practices, administrators may find themselves responsible not only for the development of a strategic plan but also for its execution. Physician leaders need to balance the demands of a busy clinical practice while also planning for the future. For successful strategic plan development and execution, ambulatory practice leaders need dedicated time to gather data, analyze, and reflect on the strategic alternatives. For the busy clinician serving in a leadership role, this may result in decreasing the number of clinic sessions for an interim period while the plan is being developed.

The practice leader must be decisive yet flexible, trustworthy, and ethical. The leader must be able to not only see the big picture but also pay attention to the details; to relate to the governing body, physicians, staff, and community leaders as well as patients. Each stakeholder group has unique perspectives and expectations of the practice. The practice leader must communicate the mission and vision of the practice while being a role model of the values. They must be a good listener and able to sort through the trivia while maintaining a focus on what is important. Keeping an eye on the future, the leader must achieve this while sustaining the viability of the current practice.

THE IMPORTANCE OF EMOTIONAL INTELLIGENCE IN HEALTHCARE LEADERSHIP

Rick Evans

Senior Vice President

Patient Services & Chief Experience Officer

New York-Presbyterian Hospital

New York, New York

When we think of leadership skills and competencies in healthcare, the list includes obvious choices: content expertise in the area of one's responsibilities, experience in leading teams, financial acumen, strategic planning prowess, project management ability, and others.

However, there is another set of skills that is sometimes overlooked (despite a lot of literature that supports it). That is *emotional intelligence*.

In more than 20 years in healthcare, I have seen leaders succeed and some fail at all levels, from managers and directors to senior-level administrators. In my experience, there is often a common thread that influences success or failure. That is whether a leader has emotional intelligence or not.

Emotional intelligence encompasses an array of abilities. First, it is connected to self-awareness. Does a leader have the ability to recognize and monitor their emotions? Are they conscious of their reactions to the situation around them? Conversely, can they "read the room" and effectively detect and respond to the reactions of others to them? Does a leader know what their trigger points might be? Self-awareness is needed for leaders to then have the ability to govern themselves in the workplace. This awareness is something that should evolve through experience and, quite honestly, often emerges from both our successes and failures.

Awareness is the foundation for another key aspect of emotional intelligence—the ability to self-regulate. Self-regulation is how we maintain professionalism and collegiality in healthcare. It allows us to consciously choose what emotions we display and express in workplace settings. It drives our personal leadership presence and professional profile. Again, in my experience, this is a major factor in leaders I have seen fail—the inability to govern themselves and their interactions. The lack of this ability degrades relationships and the willingness of others to collaborate. All too often, leaders who cannot effectively regulate themselves end up isolated. This severely inhibits their ability to get things done or to collaborate successfully.

Emotional intelligence is not only a set of skills; it is also an orientation. Leaders with emotional intelligence know that relationships are the means to achieve objectives. They are the currency of leadership and achievement. Leaders who are oriented toward building relationships cultivate them through collaboration and work actively to maintain them in times of conflict. Emotional intelligence is also an orientation toward empathy. Empathy in leadership reflects a desire to understand the needs, goals, and situations of others with whom we need to work to succeed. It acknowledges the need to create "win/win" scenarios whenever possible. When people feel you care about them and their agendas, they are more likely to be there for you when you need them in return. I've often reflected in my career on the concept of "you reap what you sow." When you demonstrate empathy and build relationships at work, you most often get the same in return. The converse is also true.

Cultivating one's emotional intelligence—both the skills and the orientation—is a key ingredient to success. No amount of clinical or administrative expertise will yield true long-term success without it. And, in its absence, difficulties will always loom. This is true even more in healthcare. Healthcare is truly a team sport. The essence of healthcare is humans serving other humans. Building emotional intelligence in leaders is consonant with healthcare's very mission. Finally, it is good for business too!

CONCLUSION

In this chapter, we discussed the important role strategic planning plays in the well-managed ambulatory practice. Having a structured, data-driven strategic planning process provides the organization with the ability to reaffirm its strategic intent. Following a defined planning process, the organization can maintain a sense of situational awareness of both the internal and external environments, consider strategic alternatives, formulate strategic goals and objectives, establish and execute an action plan, and evaluate progress towards the desired outcomes. The strategic planning process as described provides the platform from which the well-managed ambulatory practice can grow and thrive.

DISCUSSION QUESTIONS

1. Why is strategic planning an important element to a well-managed ambulatory practice?

2. Describe potential pitfalls or challenges with each step of the strategic planning process that ambulatory practice leaders should consider. Propose ways to avoid or mitigate the impact of the challenges identified.

3. Describe the elements of a PEST analysis and how the results may inform the strategic planning process.

4. Explain the notion of organizational competencies and the relevance of this concept to building organizational capacity.

5. Explain the purpose of the vision, mission, and values in the strategic planning process.

6. In reference to Figure 2.2, select any one of the pillars and discuss how it relates to the strategic intent of the ambulatory practice.

7. Explain why "do nothing" may be a viable strategic alternative when developing the list of strategic alternatives.

8. Of the four critical abilities of ambulatory practice leaders as it relates to strategy development (collaboration, team building, change leadership, and focus), select which ability you think is most important. Justify your choice.

REFERENCES

Drucker, P. F. (1994, September/October). The theory of the business. *Harvard Business Review, 72*(5), 95–104.

Drucker, P. F. (2000). *The Essential Drucker: The best of sixty years of Peter Drucker's essential writings on management.* Routledge.

Edmondson, A. C., & Lei, Z. (2014). Psychological safety: The history, renaissance, and future of an interpersonal construct. *Annual Review of Organizational Psychology and Organizational Behavior, 1*(1), 23–43.

Glenn, J. C. (2009). *Futures wheel, futures research methodology version* 3.0. Millennium Project.

Hines, A., & Bishop, P. (2015). *Thinking about the future: Guidelines for strategic foresight.* HPB.

Ibarra, H., & Hansen, M. T. (2011). Are you a collaborative leader? *Harvard Business Review, 89*(7–8), 68–74, 164.

Levi, D., & Askay, D. (2020). *Group dynamics for teams* (6th ed.) Sage.

Mankins, M., & Steele, R. (2005, July/August). Turning great strategy into great performance. *Harvard Business Review, 83*(7/8), 64–72.

Orlikoff, J. E., & Totten, M. K. (2006, July). Strategic planning: Maximizing the Board's impact. *Trustee, 59*(7), 15–20.

Prahalad, C. K., & Hamel, G. (1990). The core competence of the corporation. *Harvard Business Review, 68*(3), 79–91.

Ulrich, D., & Smallwood, N. (2004, June). Capitalizing on capabilities. *Harvard Business Review, 82*(6), 119–127.

Walston, S. L. (2013). *Strategic healthcare management: Planning and execution.* Health Administration Press.

ORGANIZATIONAL STRUCTURE

CAROL K. LUCAS

LEARNING OBJECTIVES

1. Determine the legal entity structures for ambulatory practices
2. Understand common ambulatory settings
3. Recognize the legal doctrines applicable to ambulatory practices: the corporate practice of medicine prohibition, **self-referral** prohibitions, and **anti-kickback statutes.**

KEY TERMS

Corporate Practice of Medicine

Shareholders

Corporation

Partnership

Limited Liability Company

Management Services Organization

Stark Law

Self-Referral

Anti-Kickback Statute

INTRODUCTION

Ambulatory practices come in a range of shapes and sizes from single-physician office practices to primary and specialty clinics to ambulatory surgery centers. The organizational structure of these practices is a function of three factors: the mission or purpose of the provider, the ownership of the ambulatory practice, and applicable legal requirements. This chapter addresses these factors and the ways in which they dictate the organizational structure of ambulatory practices.

In brief, although there is overlap among the factors, they can be described as follows:

- The basic determinants of organizational structure are the services that are offered by the practice. For example, will the practice offer medical services, behavioral health services, surgical services, or ancillary services? Is the practice intended to be for-profit or nonprofit?

■ Ownership frequently informs organizational structure, especially in the **corporate practice of medicine** states: Are physicians the owners, or will there be hospital or health system ownership? Is the ambulatory practice owned, in whole or in part, by investors?

■ Legal requirements are largely a matter of state law because healthcare licensing laws and regulation of healthcare practice are issues governed on a state level. Because the United States has a federal system, there is also an overlay of federal law requirements, largely but not exclusively tied to federal healthcare programs, such as Medicare. For organizational purposes, the most significant threshold question is whether the state prohibits the corporate practice of medicine, that is, whether unlicensed persons or entities are prohibited from providing healthcare services to the public. Legal requirements also address such questions as certificates of need, provider ownership of ancillary services, the regulation of self-referral, fee-splitting laws, and the like.

LEGAL ORGANIZATION

Most businesses in the United States are organized as one of three categories of entities: **partnerships**, **corporations**, or **limited liability companies**. Sole proprietorships, in contrast, operate without a legal entity structure but instead are operated by a single individual. Sole proprietorships are less common in healthcare than in other industries because of liability concerns; interposing a legal entity structure can protect owners from liability for the business, and liability has historically been a significant concern in healthcare.

Partnerships

Partnerships are business entities consisting of at least two individuals who join together for a common business purpose. Legally, they can be general partnerships or limited partnerships.

General Partnerships

In general partnerships, each partner has unlimited liability for the obligations of the partnership, and for this reason, partnerships in healthcare may be composed of partners that are themselves corporations. General partnerships may be formed without the formality of filings with the state and are based on an agreement of the partners, which may be written or oral.

All partners in a general partnership participate in the conduct of the business and share in the profits, although not necessarily equally. A written partnership agreement generally sets forth the agreements among the partners with respect to (a) the partners' respective responsibilities with respect to the business, (b) the partners' participation in management and voting rights, (c) the partners' compensation, (d) buy/sell rights, and (e) the withdrawal or expulsion of partners.

Limited Partnerships

Limited partnerships consist of at least one general partner and at least one limited partner. The general partner has the responsibility and authority to operate the business and unlimited liability for the obligations of the business. Limited partners do not participate in management (with the exception of a vote on certain fundamental decisions) and do not have liability for the obligations of the business. A limited partner can lose the investment in the partnership but is not liable beyond that (although they retain liability for their own actions). Limited partnerships are formed by filing with the state on a prescribed form.

Corporations

Corporations are legal entities separate from their owners and are considered separate legal persons, even when they are owned by a single shareholder. They are formed by filing articles or certificates of incorporation with the state. Corporations have a well-defined management structure: A board of directors has the ultimate responsibility for the management and direction of the corporation and is elected or appointed by the shareholder(s). The directors appoint the officers who report to the board.

Corporations are governed by bylaws, which set forth the size of the board of directors; determine how vacancies on the board are to be filled; establish committees of the board; delineate the responsibilities of officers of the corporation; set forth requirements for meetings of directors and **shareholders**; provide for indemnification of directors, officers, and other agents; and detail record and reporting requirements.

Corporations that have multiple shareholders active in the business, such as most medical practices organized as corporations, frequently also have shareholders' agreements that address many of the same issues that would be addressed in a partnership agreement, including the shareholders' (a) responsibilities with respective to the business; (b) participation in management and voting rights; (c) compensation; (d) buy/sell rights, and (e) withdrawal or expulsion, especially upon events that impair a shareholder's ability to participate in the business, including death, disability, loss of license, loss of staff privileges, or exclusion from federal healthcare programs.

The board of directors appoints the officers (president or chief executive officer, treasurer or chief financial officer, and secretary) who report to the board and are responsible for carrying out the directives of the board. Corporate shareholders, directors, and officers generally do not have liability for the obligations of the corporation (although they retain liability for their own actions). There are three types of corporations: general business, professional, and nonprofit.

General Business Corporations

General business corporations may engage in any lawful business other than specialized types of business, such as banking or the practice of most professions. In some states, general business corporations may engage in the practice of medicine. General business corporations are also a common entity form for ambulatory settings that do not practice medicine per se, such as ambulatory surgery centers.

Professional Corporations

Professional corporations are corporations specifically authorized for the practice of a profession, such as medicine, dentistry, and physical therapy, among others, and are the predominant form of business organization for medical practices in the United States. In many states, professions may only be practiced through a professional corporation and not a general business corporation. Even states that do not require professions to be practiced through a professional corporation permit professionals to form them and prescribe the requirements for shareholders, officers, directors, and professional employees; in those states, professional corporation statutes authorize and regulate professional corporations.

Professional corporation laws require that all or a designated percentage of shareholders, directors, and officers be licensed professionals. Shares of a professional corporation generally may not be owned by nonlicensed persons, so the shares may not be transferred by will or intestate succession (unless the transferee/heir is also licensed). Professional corporation statutes generally provide a period of three to six months for shares to be transferred into the hands of a licensed person following death or loss of license before the corporation ceases to be legally able to practice the profession for which it was organized.

Except for specific requirements related to the practice of the licensed profession, professional corporations are governed by the general corporation law in the state in which they are organized.

Nonprofit Corporations

Nonprofit corporations are a third type of corporate entity. Unlike general business corporations or professional corporations, they are organized for particular charitable, religious, educational, or another public benefit purpose. Many hospitals and health systems are organized as nonprofit entities, and in the ambulatory sector, community health centers are generally nonprofit entities.

Nonprofit corporations do not have shareholders; they are managed and operated by a board of directors and have specific restrictions on private benefit (often referred to as inurement) as a result of their tax-exempt status. If a nonprofit corporation applies for and receives designation as a tax-exempt organization from the Internal Revenue Service, it may accept tax-exempt donations of money or property.

Limited Liability Companies

Limited liability companies (LLCs) are legally a hybrid of the corporate and partnership forms in that they have the liability protection feature of corporations with the management flexibility of partnerships. Like corporations, they are formed by filing formation documents with the state. Owners of LLCs are members, rather than shareholders, and the LLC itself may be manager-managed or member-managed. LLCs, like partnerships, are pass-through entities for tax purposes. Some states have created professional limited liability companies for the practice of professions in LLC form.

The governing document of an LLC is the operating agreement or LLC agreement. The operating agreement functions as a combination of bylaws and the shareholders' agreement in the corporate setting. The operating agreement includes provisions related to meeting notice and quorum requirements, record and report requirements, and the identification of officers, as well as addressing members' responsibilities with respect to the business, members' rights to share in profits, and limitation on the power of the manager(s) to make decisions regarding the business or the company.

If the LLC is member-managed, all members participate in the business. Many LLCs are single-manager-managed, and the manager effectively functions as a combination of a corporate director and chief executive officer, with any limitations on the manager's unilateral authority spelled out in the operating agreement.

LLCs are a common business entity form for joint ventures, and in those instances, they are frequently managed by multiple managers who function similarly to a corporate board of directors. The operating agreement of such an entity generally specifies the rights of each venturer to participate in decision-making, supermajority voting requirements for any or all decisions, transfer restrictions, rights of first refusal, non-competition agreements, the redemption of members, and exit strategies.

AMBULATORY SETTINGS AND SERVICES

Healthcare in the United States is increasingly delivered in an ambulatory setting. These settings include the following.

Hospital Outpatient Departments

Hospital outpatient departments are a way for hospitals to treat patients that do not require an overnight inpatient stay. They are part of the hospital and are licensed to operate as a component of the hospital's license. The hospital bills for the services and the patients are considered hospital patients. The services range from primary care or specialty medical care to occupational or speech therapy to ambulatory surgery. Frequently, the costs are higher for hospital-based ambulatory services compared to private medical offices, in part because hospitals have significantly higher costs than most other ambulatory settings.

Private Physician Office or Clinic

Physician-owned settings vary from the small physician group practice, either primary care or specialty, to large multispecialty clinics. They are for-profit and organized as general business corporations, professional corporations, or LLCs, depending on state law. The term *clinic* may be used technically to refer to a health-care setting that operates under a specific license, such as a dialysis clinic or a rehabilitation clinic, or generically to refer to any practice that offers physician services. Urgent care clinics, for example, are physician practices under state law; the term *urgent care* is used to connote extended hours and walk-in services, but they are legally equivalent to a physician's office.

Freestanding Emergency Departments

A freestanding emergency department is a licensed facility separate from a hospital. Hospitals operate them as outpatient departments, sometimes called satellite departments, but they may also be operated by private parties. They are required to be open 24 hours per day and to have physicians present at all times. Not all states currently license non-hospital-affiliated emergency departments, and Medicare does not recognize them as emergency departments, which limits their reimbursement.

Ambulatory Surgery Centers

Ambulatory surgery centers (ASCs) are facilities that provide surgeries that do not require a stay longer than 23.5 hours by the patient. The Centers for Medicare and Medicaid Services (CMS) maintains a list of procedures that it considers appropriate for the ASC setting, and procedures are added as technological advances permit them to be done safely without a hospital stay. In terms of cost, ASCs are generally lower cost providers than hospitals because ASC overhead is generally lower.

Convenience Clinics

Convenience clinic is a term used to describe a limited primary care clinic located in a non-healthcare setting, often a retail setting such as a drug store or a grocery store. Convenience clinics are generally staffed by advanced practice providers rather than physicians. The clinics provide services on a walk-in basis to treat nonemergency healthcare needs such as simple wounds or sprains, inoculations, or illnesses. These clinics generally are not subject to licensure and operate as provider offices within the scope of practice and supervision requirements applicable to their clinical staff.

Community Health Centers

Community health centers are operated by nonprofit, tax-exempt organizations. They offer care to medically underserved populations on a free or reduced-fee basis. A subset of community health centers are Federally Qualified Health Centers (FQHCs), which are so designated by the Health Resources and Services Administration, an agency of the U.S. Department of Health and Human Services. FQHCs deliver primary care in medically underserved areas and are eligible for grant funding to assist in their mission. They may offer some specialty services as well, including dental care and behavioral healthcare. They have specific governance requirements and provide care on a sliding-fee basis depending on a patient's ability to pay.

Ancillary Care Providers

Numerous ancillary care providers, such as physical therapists, speech pathologists, and psychologists, operate on a freestanding outpatient basis. These providers generally are not subject to licensure and operate as provider offices.

IMPACT OF LEGAL REQUIREMENTS

Because healthcare is a highly regulated industry, several legal doctrines affect the organizational structure of ambulatory practices. Among these, the most significant are the corporate practice of medicine prohibition, self-referral prohibitions, and anti-kickback statutes (AKSs).

Corporate Practice of Medicine Prohibition

Many states have some form of corporate practice of medicine prohibition, which, broadly speaking, prohibits unlicensed persons from providing medical services to the public. The prohibition arose in the first half of the 20th century and was intended to protect the exercise of professional judgment from lay interference,

especially in the service of business profit. The corporate practice states have varying levels of enforcement and different exceptions to the prohibition. At its most
far-reaching, the corporate practice of medicine ban prohibits the employment
of physicians by general business corporations and even by hospitals (American
Health Lawyers' Association, 2020).

The ban does not apply to appropriately constituted professional corporations but
to entities owned and operated by nonlicensees. In most states, professional corporations must be wholly owned by licensed persons, and licensed persons must
be the directors and officers of the entity. Exceptions exist in some states for the
employment of physicians by hospitals, licensed clinics, nonprofit entities, and
government-run healthcare providers.

In states that prohibit the corporate practice of medicine, lay investors in healthcare businesses have developed a **management services organization** (MSO)/friendly
professional corporation (PC) model. Under this model, an MSO, owned wholly or in
part by non-licensed individuals, provides administrative support services to a practice pursuant to a written services agreement. Often, the MSO provides everything
that does not require a medical license, including space, supplies, equipment, nonprofessional staff, accounting, billing and collection, and payables management. A well-
crafted management services agreement clearly recognizes the corporation's control
over all clinical decisions and the practice itself, including the authority to hire physicians, set clinical protocols, and enter into agreements to provide medical services.

The MSO/friendly PC model permits physicians to concentrate on the practice of medicine while delegating to experienced managers the myriad nonclinical
functions necessary to maintain financial stability. It also provides a vehicle for
investment capital, by providing a mechanism for unlicensed investors to provide
financing to medical businesses. For this reason, most telemedicine businesses are
organized using the MSO/friendly PC model, as are specialty practices requiring
expensive equipment, such as vascular access centers or radiation oncology practices. The model further permits practices to realize economies of scale by pooling
support resources while maintaining control over their individual practices. In this
respect, the MSO/friendly PC model functions as a species of a joint venture, governed by a services agreement rather than existing as a single legal entity such as
an LLC.

The corporate practice prohibition affects a large number of disparate ambulatory practices. For example, in corporate practice states, lay entities are prohibited from owning urgent care clinics, so any urgent care practice that involves
nonlicensed investors must be set up using the MSO/friendly PC model. The
management services agreement between the entities generally specifies that the
professional corporation will have complete authority and responsibility over clinical matters, while the MSO provides support, including space, nonprofessional
staff, supplies, equipment, third-party services, and so on. The agreement may also

give the MSO the right to designate a successor holder of the corporation stock in order to protect the substantial investment made by the lay investors.

The MSO is usually tasked with marketing and branding the practice. Extreme care must be taken in advertising; most states regulate physician advertising, and any copy that suggests that the MSO is providing medical services potentially puts both the MSO and the professional corporation owner at legal risk. Should the MSO be deemed to exercise excessive control over the practice of medicine, it can be prosecuted for the unlicensed practice of medicine and the physician affiliated with it may face licensure action for unprofessional conduct or even prosecution for aiding and abetting the unlicensed practice of medicine.

The corporate practice ban also affects the way that payments for medical services are handled. In a corporate practice state, payment for medical services must be made to the professional corporation, not to the MSO, because the professional corporation is the entity providing the medical services. The management company generally has access to the corporation's operating account in order to fulfill its services responsibilities, including payroll oversight and payables management, but may only access funds itself in the form of its services fee. Most management services agreements provide that if there is insufficient revenue to pay professional expenses (i.e., clinician compensation) and the management fee, the management fee will be deferred, as necessary.

The prohibition on direct employment of physicians affects almost every ambulatory practice in corporate practice states. Convenience clinics, for example, in corporate practice states cannot be directly operated by the retail business in which they are located. Rather, clinics, even if staffed only by nurse practitioners, must be owned by a professional corporation and managed by the retailer or a third party. The corporate practice ban also complicates arrangements with entities such as accountable care organizations and medical foundations because it requires participation by a freestanding physician entity rather than permitting direct employment of the physicians.

Self-Referral Prohibitions

The **Stark Law** prohibits physicians from referring patients for designated health services that will be billed to Medicare or another federal healthcare program to an entity if the physician (or an immediate family member) has a financial relationship with the entity.[1] Designated health services are clinical laboratory services; physical therapy, occupational therapy, and speech language pathology services; radiology and certain other imaging services; radiation therapy service and supplies; durable

---

[1] 42 USC § 1395nn.

medical equipment; parenteral and enteral nutrients; prosthetic orthotics and prosthetic devices; home health services; outpatient prescription drugs; and inpatient and outpatient hospital services. Note that outpatient surgery is not a designated health service, a circumstance that has fostered physician investment in ambulatory surgery centers. On the other hand, inpatient and outpatient hospital services are designated health services, which means that any ambulatory setting or financial relationship that involves a hospital and physicians on its medical staff requires a Stark analysis.

A financial relationship can be either an ownership interest or a compensation relationship and includes indirect as well as direct relationships. A violation of the Stark Law could lead to overpayment and refund requirements, False Claims Act liability,[2] program exclusions for knowing violations, civil monetary penalties up to $15,000 for each service and/or $100,000 for each arrangement considered to be a circumvention scheme, and damages of up to three times the amount billed to the federal healthcare program.

Violation of the Stark Law does not require proof of intent. Any prohibited referral, no matter how innocent, constitutes a violation unless it satisfies all the elements of an exception to the Stark Law.

Because a financial relationship may be either an ownership interest or a compensation relationship, almost any ambulatory practice that involves physicians and services that will be billed to Medicare or another federal healthcare program can only be structured with reference to the Stark Law. Any services relationship between a physician or group of physicians, on one hand, and a hospital or other provider of designated health services, on the other hand, requires an analysis of the compensation relationship between the parties. The most common Stark Law exceptions relevant to physician–hospital arrangements are those relating to personal services arrangements, leases of space and equipment, and in-office ancillary services, each of which contains specific requirements that must be satisfied in order to avoid a violation of the Stark Law. Thus, any physician services relationship with a hospital outpatient department, such as a medical directorship, for example, is required to satisfy the terms of the personal services exception.

Personal Services Exception

Under the personal services exception, a personal services arrangement does not constitute a financial relationship, if all the following conditions are met:[3]

1. Each arrangement is set out in writing, is signed by the parties, and specifies the services covered by the arrangement.

---

[2] 31 USC §§ 3729-3733.
[3] 42 CFR 411.357(d)(1).

2. The arrangement(s) covers all services to be furnished by the physician (or an immediate family member of the physician) to the entity. This requirement is met if all separate arrangements between the entity and the physician and the entity and any family members incorporate each other by reference or if they cross-reference a master list of contracts maintained and updated centrally and is available for review by the Secretary of Health and Human Services upon request. The master list must be maintained in a manner that preserves the historical record of contracts. A physician or family member can "furnish" services through employees whom they have hired for the purpose of performing the services, through a wholly owned entity, or through locum tenens physicians (as defined at §411.351 of this subpart, except that the regular physician need not be a member of a group practice).

3. The aggregate services for which are contracted do not exceed those that are reasonable and necessary for the legitimate business purposes of the arrangement(s).

4. The term of each arrangement is for at least one year. To meet this requirement, if an arrangement is terminated during the term with or without cause, the parties may not enter into the same or substantially the same arrangement during the first year of the original term of the arrangement.

5. The compensation to be paid over the term of each arrangement is set in advance, does not exceed fair market value, and, except in the case of a physician incentive plan (as defined at §411.351 of this subpart), is not determined in a manner that takes into account the volume or value of any referrals or other business generated between the parties.

6. The services to be furnished under each arrangement do not involve the counseling or promotion of a business arrangement or other activity that violates any federal or state law.

Rental of Space and Equipment Exception

Similarly, any lease between a physician and a hospital requires reference to the Stark exception for space leases to include a physician's practice in a medical office building owned by the hospital.[4] The lease exception provides that payments for use of office space made by a lessee to a lessor do not constitute a prohibited financial relationship if the arrangement meets the following requirements:

1. The lease arrangement is set out in writing, is signed by the parties, and specifies the premises it covers.

2. The duration of the lease arrangement is at least one year.

---

[4] 42 USC §1395nn(e)(1).

3. The space rented or leased does not exceed that which is reasonable and necessary for the legitimate business purpose of the lease arrangement and is used exclusively by the lessee (when being used by the lessee) and is not shared with or used by the lessor.

4. The rental charges over the term of the lease arrangement are set in advance and are consistent with fair market value,

5. The rental charges over the term of the lease arrangement are not determined in any manner that takes into account the volume or value of referrals or other business generated between the parties.

6. The lease arrangement would be commercially reasonable even if no referrals were made between the lessee and the lessor.

The Stark exception for equipment leases is similar to that for space leases: Equipment leases must be in writing, signed by the parties, for a term of at least one year, and the rental must be set in advance and consistent with fair market value.

The Stark compensation exceptions depend on the compensation being commensurate with fair market value because if compensation for services or rent paid for space or equipment represents fair market value, no portion of the payment is payment for the referral of patients, and the relationship is bona fide. Determination of fair market value frequently requires an independent third-party valuation expert to validate the compensation or lease rate if the Stark Law is implicated by a particular relationship.

In-Office Ancillary Services Exception

For the purposes of structuring ambulatory practices, however, the Stark prohibition on physician referrals to entities in which they have an ownership interest is much more significant than that applicable to compensation relationships.[5] Any ambulatory clinic that includes its own laboratory or imaging service, or that provides physical or occupational therapy, must be mindful of the Stark Law and the requirements of the in-office ancillary services exception.

The in-office ancillary services exception to the Stark Law allows a physician to refer a patient for designated health services to the physician's own office or the office of the physician's "group practice" if certain criteria are met. These criteria are known as the "supervision," "billing," and "location" requirements. In addition, the premise of the discussion is the qualification of the referring physician's group as a "group practice" for the purposes of the Stark Law.

The supervision requirement. Under the supervision requirement,[6] the designated health services must be furnished personally by the referring physician,

---

[5] 42 USC § 1395nn(b)(2).
[6] 42 CFR § 411.355(b)(1)(iii).

a physician who is a member of the referring physician's group practice, or an individual who is supervised by the referring physician or another physician who is "in the same group practice." To be a physician who is "in the same group practice," the supervising physician can be, among other things, an owner, an employee, or an independent contractor of the group practice. For example, a physician could refer patients to the practice's own in-house provider of a designated health service if the services are performed by the practice's ancillary personnel who are supervised by a physician employed or contracted by the practice. The physician's supervision of ancillary personnel must be consistent with the level required by the applicable Medicare billing and payment rules.

The billing requirement. Under the billing requirement,[7] the designated health services must be billed by either the physician who supervises the service or the group practice in which the supervising physician is a physician. The services may also be billed by an entity that is wholly owned by the group practice.

The location requirement. Under the location requirement,[8] the designated health services must be furnished in the same building as the group practice maintains its offices or a centralized location.

For purposes of the in-office ancillary services exception, the ambulatory practice must be a "group practice" as defined by the Stark Law.[9] Among other requirements of a group practice under Stark, each physician who is a member of the group must furnish "substantially the full range of patient care services that the physician routinely furnishes, including medical care, consultation, diagnosis, and treatment, through the joint use of shared office space, facilities, equipment and personnel." The so-called substantially all test means that at least 75% of the total patient care services of the group's physician owners and employees must be furnished through the group and billed under a billing number assigned to the group. Stark defines *patient care services* as including not only direct patient treatment but also performing administrative or management-related tasks.

As an example, assume that the group practice has three owners, one who provides 100% of his patient care services each week through the group and two others two who provide 10%. Furthermore, assume that the group practice employs 10 physicians who each provide an average of 90% of their routine physician services each week to the group.

---

[7] 42 CFR § 411.355(b)(3).
[8] 42 CFR § 411.355(b)(2).
[9] 42 CFR § 411.352.

$$2 \text{ physician owners at } 10\% \text{ each} = 20\%$$

$$1 \text{ owner at } 100\% = 100\%$$

$$10 \text{ employed physicians at } 90\% \text{ each} = 900\%$$

$$1020\% \text{ divided by } 13 \text{ physicians} = 78.46\% \text{ average}$$

In this scenario, 78.46% of the patient care services provided by the group's share-holders and physician employees are provided through the group, which exceeds the substantially all test's 75% threshold.

Another component of the Stark Law's definition of *group practice* is the so-called patient-encounters test. This test requires members of the group, that is, partners or employees, to personally conduct at least 75% of the group's physician–patient encounters.[10] An *encounter* is any appointment during which a patient is examined or treated by a physician.[11] This test measures patient encounters on a per capita basis, not in units of time.

To illustrate how the patient-encounters test works, consider the following scenario: Three part-time physician independent contractors collectively conduct an average of 150 physician–patient encounters each week for the group. The group's three owners provide 100 patient encounters on average each week (with two of the owners providing none). Three physician employees conduct 150 patient encounters on average each week for the group. Under this scenario, members of the group, that is, partners and employees but not independent contractors, would conduct 250 (100 + 150) of the total 400 (150 + 100 + 150), or 62.5%, of the group's patient encounters. Such an arrangement would fail the 75% patient-encounter threshold, and the practice therefore would not constitute a group practice for Stark Law purposes.

The remaining elements of the Stark definition of *group practice* require the group to be a "unified business" with centralized decision-making, a pooling of expenses and revenues, and a method of compensation and profit distribution not based on satellite offices operating as if they are separate enterprises or profit centers.[12] In addition, no physician who is a member of the group can directly or indirectly receive compensation based on the volume or value of that physician's referrals, with an exception for productivity bonuses having prescribed parameters.[13]

In order to determine whether the Stark law affects the structure of a particular ambulatory setting the following decision tree should be applied: First, does the

---

[10] 42 CFR § 411.352(h).
[11] 63 Fed. Reg. 1659, 1690 (Jan. 9, 1998).
[12] 42 CFR § 411.352(f).
[13] 42 CFR § 411.352(g).

ambulatory practice involve physicians? If so, will the ambulatory practice provide services that will be billed to Medicare or another federal healthcare program? If so, will the ambulatory practice offer a designated health service (i.e., imaging, lab, physical therapy, durable medical equipment, etc.)? If the answer to all of these questions is yes, the inquiry shifts to whether the ambulatory practice satisfies the *group practice* definition under Stark. If any of the first three questions is answered in the negative (i.e., there will be no physician referrals, no billing to a federal healthcare program, or no designated health service), then the Stark analysis may stop and no review of the group practice definition is required.

Even if a particular ambulatory setting is not required to comply with the Stark Law, it is important to note that many states have analogous self-referral laws. Further complicating the structuring of an ambulatory practice, however, is the fact that not all state self-referral laws track the Stark Law perfectly. They may apply to different ancillary services, for example, or use a different definition for services provided within a physician's own practice.

Anti-Kickback Statutes

The Stark Law prohibits self-referral by physicians. The federal AKS[14] prohibits payment or acceptance of payment for referrals by any person if the service will be billed to the Medicare program or another federal healthcare program. Therefore, the AKS can be applicable even if no physician is involved and if no designated health services are provided. Both statutes are intended to protect the integrity of the Medicare program, but their focuses, and therefore their reach, are somewhat different.

The AKS establishes criminal penalties for individuals or entities who knowingly and willfully offer, pay, solicit, or receive remuneration in order to compensate or induce referrals of business that are reimbursable under Medicare or any other federal healthcare program.[15] In theory, payments by an ambulatory practice to its owners for their ownership interests in in the practice, including the ancillary services offered by the practice, could be construed as payments for the physicians' referrals to the practice. Because the AKS is a criminal statute, intent is required to establish a violation.

The AKS provides several safe harbors. These safe harbors operate somewhat differently from the Stark exceptions. Under the Stark Law, if an arrangement fails to satisfy every element of the applicable exception, the Stark Law is violated. The AKS safe harbors, on the other hand, establish minimum standards that arrangements

---

[14] 42 USC §1320a-7b.
[15] 42 USC §1320a-7b(b)(1)-(2).

can meet in order to avoid prosecution for a kickback violation. Although the satisfaction of all the elements of a safe harbor will shield an arrangement from AKS liability, the converse is not true. The fact that a particular arrangement fails to satisfy every element of the applicable safe harbor does not mean that a violation of the AKS has occurred. The violation still requires an intentional payment or acceptance of payment for a referral.

The AKS has a safe harbor for investment in a group practice.[16] This safe harbor permits owners to earn a return on their investment in the group practice, such as dividend income, if the following tests are met:

1. The equity interests in the group practice are held by licensed healthcare professionals who practice in the group.

2. The equity interests in the group are held in the group itself, as distinguished from any subdivision of the group.

3. The group satisfies the Stark definition of *group practice* set forth in the Stark statute.

4. Revenues from ancillary services are derived from in-office ancillary services that meet the definition of that term under Stark.

It is notable that the AKS safe harbor for investment in a group practice imports the Stark definitions of *group practice* and *in-office ancillary services*.

The AKS also provides a safe harbor for personal services arrangements[17] that tracks the Stark Law exception for personal services arrangements in many respects. Under the personal services safe harbor, *remuneration* does not include any payment made by a principal (the ambulatory practice) to an agent (a service provider, e.g., a physician) as compensation for the services of the agent, as long as all of the following seven standards are met:

1. The agency agreement is set out in writing and signed by the parties.

2. The agency agreement covers all the services the agent provides to the principal for the term of the agreement and specifies the services to be provided by the agent.

3. If the agency agreement is intended to provide for the services of the agent on a periodic, sporadic, or part-time basis, rather than on a full-time basis, for the term of the agreement, the agreement specifies exactly the schedule of such intervals, their precise length, and the exact charge for such intervals.

4. The term of the agreement is for not less than one year.

---

[16] 42 CFR §1001.952(p).
[17] 42 CFR §1001.952(d).

5. The aggregate compensation paid to the agent over the term of the agreement is set in advance, is consistent with fair market value in arm's-length transactions, and is not determined in a manner that takes into account the volume or value of any referrals or business otherwise generated between the parties for which payment may be made in whole or in part under Medicare or other federal healthcare programs.

6. The services performed under the agreement do not involve the counseling or promotion of a business arrangement or other activity that violates any state or federal law.

7. The aggregate services contracted for do not exceed those which are reasonably necessary to accomplish the commercially reasonable business purpose of the services.

INTEGRATION OF AMBULATORY PRACTICES WITH OTHER ENTITIES

Unlike models in other countries that feature a government-sponsored or government-run healthcare system, the healthcare system in the United States is inherently entrepreneurial and fragmented. Increasingly, however, the healthcare system is focusing on integrated or coordinated care to promote both efficiency and better patient outcomes. Models like the accountable care organization (ACO) and the patient-centered medical home (PCMH) are entities intended to coordinate care among disparate providers, including hospitals, physicians, and other healthcare providers, but structuring them remains subject to state and federal laws.

Accountable Care Organizations

ACOs were introduced in the Affordable Care Act in 2010. An ACO is a healthcare delivery model in which a group of physicians, hospitals, and other healthcare providers work together to coordinate care for people enrolled in Medicare. The participants in the ACO agree to share responsibility for the quality, cost, and coordination of care with aligned incentives for a defined population of patients. The ACO uses the fee-for-service payment system of original Medicare program but provides financial incentives to participants to control costs.

ACOs under the Affordable Care Act are limited to services provided to enrollees in the traditional fee-for-service Medicare. Alongside those ACOs, however, many private-sector health insurers have adopted the model, often referred to as a "commercial ACO," which may be offered through a health maintenance organization or preferred provider organization plan. Commercial ACOs frequently rely on tiered or narrow networks as a way to control costs by negotiating favorable rates from providers who anticipate patient volume or by excluding providers seen as high cost.

Patient-Centered Medical Home

PCMH is a primary care model built on a direct relationship between a patient and a particular provider that coordinates a team of collaborating healthcare professionals to provide comprehensive care. The medical home is accountable for meeting a substantial portion of each patient's physical and mental health care needs, including prevention and wellness, acute care, and chronic care. Providing comprehensive care involves a team of care providers, including physicians, advanced practice nurses, nurses, pharmacists, nutritionists, social workers, and care coordinators. The team may be part of a single practice or may work together across a number of practice settings.

Ambulatory practices engaged in ACOs and PCMHs remain subject to the legal requirements described earlier: In corporate practice of medicine states, the practice must be organized as an independent professional organization; the Stark Law affects the practice's ability to offer ancillary services, such as laboratory or imaging services, and to engage in financial relationships with hospitals and other providers of designated health services; and the AKS affects the practice's financial relationships with any party with which it has a referral relationship.

Evolving delivery models aim to improve cost and quality by increasing coordination of providers, and all include ambulatory practices. Despite the novelty of the entity, they remain subject to complying with federal and state law regarding their organization and structure.

CONCLUSION

Ambulatory practices are the building blocks of healthcare delivery in the United States. Their legal organization depends on several factors, including the services they offer, their ownership, and the legal and payer requirements applicable to them. In addition, because the United States has a federal legal system, most ambulatory practices are subject to an overlapping network of state and federal requirements. State law governs legal organization and licensure, while the federal Medicare program, as the largest payer in the United States, imposes its own requirements that determine the structure of ambulatory practices and the ways in which they can coordinate with each other.

DISCUSSION QUESTIONS

1. What are the legal entity structures that are common for ambulatory practices? What are the considerations in selecting a structure?

2. You are the manager of a new ambulatory practice, and one of the physicians asks you about installing a CT scanner to which to refer patients for imaging. What law should you reference to learn more about action steps?

3. Describe the four tests for investment in a group practice as defined by the safe harbor of the Anti-Kickback statute. Explain the relevance of the test for a group of physicians.

4. Describe the basic tenets of the Stark Law and how it may impact an ambulatory practice.

REFERENCE

American Health Lawyers' Association. (2020). *Corporate practice of medicine: A 50 state survey* (2nd ed.).

QUALITY, SAFETY, AND PATIENT EXPERIENCE

WITH CONTRIBUTING AUTHOR KRISTIN BAIRD

LEARNING OBJECTIVES

1. Explain the national policies and advocacy efforts to improve quality, safety, and patient experience

2. Identify organizational structures and processes designed to improve quality, safety, and experience in the ambulatory setting

3. Describe the tools and strategies designed to increase the use of evidence-based interventions in performance improvement initiatives

4. Recognize the role of patient experience in evaluating quality of care

KEY TERMS

Institute of Medicine

Outcomes

Donabedian Model

Ambulatory Care Sensitive Conditions

Patient-Reported Outcome Measures

Latent Conditions

Triple Aim

Journey Map

Process Improvement

INTRODUCTION

The well-managed ambulatory practice necessitates administrators who understand and prioritize the continuous improvement of quality, safety, and patient experience. "Safe, high-quality ambulatory care requires complex information management and care coordination across multiple settings," according to the Agency for Healthcare Research and Quality (AHRQ, 2018). The heterogeneous nature of the ambulatory care setting presents unique challenges to measure, monitor, and improve these vital elements. For these reasons, the manager must be skilled in understanding the subject matter as well as the improvement tools that can serve as resources to support endeavors to enhance quality, safety, and patient experience.

QUALITY

The **Institute of Medicine** (IOM, 1990) defines *healthcare quality* as "the degree to which health care services for individuals and populations increase the likelihood of desired health **outcomes** and are consistent with current professional knowledge." Figure 4.1 outlines the six domains of quality, according to the IOM.

The definition of *quality* has evolved over time (see Exhibit 4.1). Different metrics, coupled with science and technology, have allowed an increasingly sophisticated inquiry into quality in the ambulatory setting. Efforts to identify and improve quality began at the turn of the 20th century in the United States. Considered the pioneer in patient outcomes, Dr. Ernest Codman, a Boston surgeon, resolved to address the lack of outcomes measurement or monitoring. Codman's systematic efforts in the 1910s, featured monitoring the progress of his patients following their treatment in order to document their results. Codman's endeavors ultimately led to the founding of the "End Result Hospital." Codman measured and categorized errors by type.

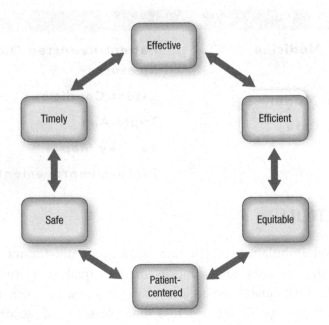

FIGURE 4.1 Quality domains.

SOURCE: Adapted from the Institute of Medicine. (2001). *Crossing the quality chasm: A new health system for the 21st century.* National Academies Press.

EXHIBIT 4.1 PIONEERS OF HEALTHCARE QUALITY AND SAFETY

1860s – Clara Barton promoted sanitary conditions to affect outcomes.

1900s – Elizabeth Blackwell recognized the differences in treatments related to the provider's gender.

1910s – Ernest Codman tracked patients to monitor and analyze outcomes.

1930s – Walter Shewhart postulated that data were influenced by their context, leading to the development of the Shewhart cycle, which is better known as the Plan–Do–Study–Act (PDSA) cycle.

1950s – Edward Deming cultivated the importance of understanding and managing variation.

1966 – Avedis Donabedian introduced a model for quality, adding outcomes to process and structure.

1967 – Alvan Feinstein focused attention on the role of clinical reasoning and identified biases that can affect it, advancing the concept of clinical judgment.

1972 – Archie Cochrane identified the lack of randomized controlled trials (RCTs) supporting many practices that had previously been assumed to be effective.

1973 – John Wennberg documented wide variations in how physicians practiced.

1980s – David Eddy described errors in clinical reasoning and gaps in evidence, advancing the concept of evidence-based medicine.

1980s – Researchers at the RAND Corporation demonstrated that large proportions of procedures performed by physicians were considered inappropriate even by the standards of their own experts.

1986 – Joseph Juran introduced the Quality Trilogy (also known as the "Juran Trilogy"), composed of quality planning, quality control, and quality improvement, that propelled the Pareto principle into use for quality improvement.

2000 – James Reason identified **latent conditions** as distinguished from active failures that lead to safety problems in healthcare.

An innovator in the now-familiar process of transparency when errors are made, Codman produced and published openly the findings of his evaluations in an annual report that allowed "patients [to] judge for themselves the quality and the outcome of care" (Neuhauser, 2002). Codman's efforts led to the initiation of the Minimum Standard for Hospitals, a one-page checklist of requirements to which hospitals were expected to adhere. In 1917, the American College of Surgeons

THE DONABEDIAN MODEL: EXPANDING YOUR KNOWLEDGE

Donabedian proposed three principal factors that combine to formulate quality: structure, process, and outcomes. Additional information about each element in the ambulatory setting is as follows:

Structure refers to all aspects describing the context in which care is delivered. This can be the setting, the providers, the personnel, and the technology involved in care delivery. For example, contrast the structure of care provided in a procedure room at an ambulatory surgery center by a trained surgeon with skilled nursing and support personnel to care rendered in a physician's office by unskilled clinical support personnel. Structure also considers population characteristics like demographics and geography that may ultimately contribute to the infrastructure of care in the given area. Structural elements are easily observable.

Process refers to all actions taken in the delivery of healthcare services. These can be administrative responsibilities, clinical duties, and even tasks attributed to the patient associated with some identified care delivery process (e.g., patients' adherence to medication instructions). A process can be technical (what one does and how they do it) or interpersonal (how one behaves or relates to others, such as the coordination of care between providers). Donabedian (2003) viewed the measurement of processes as closely approximating the quality of care. For example, perhaps concern has been raised about misidentified blood specimens collected in the ambulatory practice's laboratory. The situation is causing clinical results to be recorded in the wrong patient's charts. The process involves a multitude of steps: the patient's initial registration, the order for blood work, the communication with the phlebotomist, the procedure to label the specimen tube, and so forth, all the way to the conclusion of the process in which results are recorded and communicated to the ordering provider. Any step of the process—or perhaps a series of them—may contribute to the results. Although processes may be observed, it's essential to comprehensively identify and understand every step in order to begin the journey to improve quality.

Outcome, according to Donabedian, refers to the "effects of healthcare." These "effects" can be on patients as well as groups of patients, or populations. Outcomes may be measured in terms of morbidity and mortality, quality of life or functional status, or other factors. They may also include patient experience. Of the three components, outcomes measurement lagged the other two in terms of focus and improvement. There are several reasons for the delay. As Donabedian noted, it is important to identify structure and process linkages to outcomes. Recognizing the connection to the observed outcome requires a thoughtful, data-driven process to establish a cause-and-effect relationship. If resources or data are limited, the inability to generate actionable findings may discourage any attempt to improve the process. Defining valid and reliable outcomes measures has proved challenging and requires sound source data, agreement on the measure, and clear evidence that the measure has acceptable sensitivity and specificity.

began to inspect hospitals for basic quality standards, which expanded over the subsequent decades.

The American College of Surgeons partnered with the American College of Physicians, the American Hospital Association, the American Medical Association, and the Canadian Medical Association to form the Joint Commission on Accreditation of Hospitals (JCAH) in 1951 (The Joint Commission [TJC], 2020). The launch of the accreditation organization established a standardized approach to healthcare quality. At the time, the organization only accredited hospitals as its name implied. Hospitals receiving JCAH accreditation, which became a condition of participation in federal programs like Medicare, were deemed to meet minimum "quality" standards. The definition of *quality*, therefore, was inferred to be the adherence to these standards. Hospitals proudly displayed their accreditation status to convey their "quality." The accrediting organization, which became the Joint Commission on Accreditation of Healthcare Organizations (JCAHO) launched an Ambulatory Health Care Accreditation program specifically aimed at quality in ambulatory practices. (The organization later went through another alteration to its title; in 2007, it was renamed the Joint Commission.)

Professional associations involved primarily in the ambulatory setting formed the Accreditation Association for Ambulatory Health Care (AAAHC) in 1979. Both accrediting organizations, along with several others that were subsequently formed, offer services to certify or recognize ambulatory practices that meet or exceed key quality standards.

Donabedian Model

Accreditation became a means for healthcare organizations to confirm their adherence to quality standards, but most of the early focus on quality standards was on the structures and processes of care. In 1966, Dr. Avedis Donabedian introduced a third component of quality—outcomes. Donabedian (2005) authored the article, "Evaluating the Quality of Medical Care," a seminal work that created a framework for quality that remains in use today. Dr. Donabedian, a physician by training, purports three foundational elements to understanding quality: structure, process, and outcome. Donabedian's premise, now referred to as the **Donabedian Model**, was that it was possible to assess the quality of care through the lenses of structure, process, and outcome. Donabedian (2003) described the calculus of quality as emanating from two factors: "the science and technology of health care" and the "application of that science and technology in actual practice." Quality, he suggested, was the "product" of these two factors. The dimensions of quality identified by Donabedian were efficacy, effectiveness, efficiency, optimality, acceptability, legitimacy, and equity (Donabedian, 2003, pp. 4–6; see the sidebar "The Donabedian Model" for more details).

By the mid-1990s, outcomes and other performance measurement data had been integrated into the process of evaluation by the accreditation organizations like TJC and the AAAHC. There was a new focus on the adherence to standards shown to link to favorable health outcomes, consistent with the model developed by Donabedian. Progress was evaluated based on performance against a set of national benchmarks and improvement from self-identified deficiencies.

Ambulatory practices continue to further efforts to improve quality through the accreditation process, internal efforts, and engagement with techniques such as lean thinking (see the sidebar "Lean Thinking in Ambulatory Practice").

Quality Measures

Every encounter in an ambulatory practice offers the opportunity to deliver high-quality care. Efforts need be both comprehensive and sustainable. Establishing, monitoring, and reporting evidence-based quality measures facilitates the

LEAN THINKING IN AMBULATORY PRACTICE

Lean thinking, which emanated from the Toyota Production System (TPS), was originally created to improve Toyota's automobile manufacturing process in Japan. The model flew in the face of car manufacturing in the United States at the time. In the United States, cars traveled down the production line until the finished product rolled off the assembly line, at which point, a team of inspectors reviewed the finished product for defects. Efforts to improve quality arrived too late to make changes and proved too expensive to toss out the finished product. Thus, many of the cars manufactured and sold in the United States were of inconsistent quality.

The TPS instead begins with the end goal in mind. What is the outcome we desire? Management then develops specifications, which are, in turn, used to construct the manufacturing process. The manufacturing process is "structured" to support the goal by having the right people, skills, and parts at the right places. "Processes" are developed and aligned according to the specifications needed to attain the desired "outcome." Instead of waiting to inspect the final product for quality, the true benefit comes from building quality into each step and empowering workers with the ability to "stop the line" if there is a deviation from specifications. As a result, only value-added processes are included in the manufacturing process, and the end product is consistently of high quality.

Ambulatory practices, along with many other sectors of healthcare, began to adopt the TPS in the early 1990s to improve the quality and efficiency of healthcare. The fundamental tenets of TPS include reducing non-value-added work (*muda*), addressing unevenness in an operation (*mura*), and minimizing the burden of equipment or employees (*muri*). The goal is to design a process capable of delivering the desired outcomes.

delivery of quality care to every patient in an ambulatory practice. **Patient-reported outcome measures** (PROMs) and **ambulatory care sensitive conditions** (ACSCs) are two examples of establishing and monitoring metrics in the ambulatory setting, aimed at improving quality.

Patient-Reported Outcome Measures

Quality of life is an important outcome of healthcare for a patient, yet it is challenging to quantify and measure. To measure a patient's ability to survive chemotherapy treatment, researchers Karnofsky and colleagues (1948) proposed a scale from 0 (for "dead") to 100 (for "normal") in 1948 for use in a clinical setting. After the introduction of the scale—referred to as the Karnofsky Performance Index—a multitude of patient-focused questionnaires regarding health status evolved. Some elaborated on the impact of illness; others on physical function or ability. Most instruments, regardless of the details, remained that which a provider reported on behalf of the patient until well into the turn of the 21st century.

Many credit the Food and Drug Administration's (FDA, 2009) embrace of patient-reported outcome measures (PROMs) as a component of clinical trials in the mid-2000s for propelling the integration of patient voice in reflecting and reporting perceptions of their outcomes as a key marker of quality. According to the FDA, "a PRO is any report of the status of a patient's health condition that comes directly from the patient, without interpretation of the patient's response by a clinician or anyone else." The FDA further elaborates: "The outcome can be measured in absolute terms (e.g., severity of a symptom, sign, or state of a disease) or as a change from a previous measure."

PROMs, often accompanied by patient-reported experience measures (PREMs), have since been embraced as critical quality measurements for ambulatory practices. Because ambulatory practices are the locations at which patients often present before and after a major treatment event, PROM and PREM surveys are commonplace. Given the bevy of information balanced with avoiding disruptions to an efficient care journey at the practice, leaders may need to determine which survey instruments to use—and how to best distribute and administer them. Technology offers an opportunity to incorporate surveys into the clinical intake process, with the integration of algorithms allowing instruments to be customized based on the patient's treatment. For example, if the patient presents to a multispecialty practice for an appointment with the neurologist, a survey focused on PROMs for neurology would be triggered if the patient was roomed for the neurologist. Survey instruments may instead be geared toward a specific demographic, complaint, treatment, or another measurement in which understanding the patient's perspective may provide value. Research in this field offers evidence-based surveys, of which results may be compared to peers to gain even deeper insight into opportunities. Regardless of the specifics, an ambulatory practice offers an excellent environment to capture the patient's voice in quality measurement. PROMs and PREMs may enhance an ambulatory practice's efforts to improve quality.

Ambulatory Care Sensitive Conditions

Data regarding quality improvement efforts in an ambulatory practice may be gleaned from another source within a healthcare system—the inpatient setting. In the early 1990s, ACSCs came to the forefront of quality improvement initiatives when researchers recognized that patients' outcomes were influenced by factors outside of the specific treatment for the condition (Billings, 1993). ACSCs are "conditions for which good outpatient care can potentially prevent the need for hospitalization, or for which early intervention can prevent complications or more severe disease" (AHRQ, 2001). ACSCs offer insight into the quality of the healthcare delivery system, as these conditions could be managed at an ambulatory practice. As examples, hospital admissions for ambulatory-sensitive conditions such as asthma, high blood pressure, or diabetes may be tracked to determine if they are possibly preventable had they been effectively treated in the ambulatory setting. See Table 4.1 for sample ACSCs.

The World Health Organization (WHO) considers ACSCs to be a key marker of performance for the healthcare system of a country: "Success in the provision of ambulatory personal health services, i.e., providing individuals with treatment for acute illness and preventive health care on an ambulatory basis, is the most significant contributor to the health care system's performance in most developing countries" (Berman, 2000). If the conditions are not effectively handled by an ambulatory

TABLE 4.1 Ambulatory Care Sensitive Conditions

CHRONIC CONDITIONS	ACUTE CONDITIONS
Diabetes short-term complications	Bacterial pneumonia
Diabetes long-term complications	Urinary tract infection
Uncontrolled diabetes	Cellulitis
Low-extremity amputation	Pressure ulcers
COPD	Dehydration
Asthma	
Hypertension	
Heart failure	

SOURCE: CMS Measures Inventory Tool. (2021, February 1). *Hospitalization for ambulatory care sensitive conditions.* https://cmit.cms.gov/CMIT_public/ReportMeasure?measureRevisionId=933

TABLE 4.2 Risk-Standardized Rates of Ambulatory Care Sensitive Hospitalizations and ED Visits, 2019

	10TH PERCENTILE (HIGH PERFORMING)	50TH PERCENTILE	90TH PERCENTILE (LOW PERFORMING)	RATIO OF 90TH TO 10TH PERCENTILE
AMBULATORY CARE SENSITIVE HOSPITALIZATIONS	35.1	48.9	66.6	1.9
AMBULATORY CARE SENSITIVE ED VISITS	62.4	98.6	150.0	2.4

SOURCE: Medicare Payment Advisory Commission. (2021, March). *Report to Congress: Medicare payment policy* (p. 114). http://medpac.gov/docs/default-source/reports/mar21_medpac_report_to_the_congress_sec.pdf

NOTE: Risk-standardized rate is expressed per 1,000 fee-for-service (FFS) beneficiaries; data was sourced using 2019 Medicare FFS claims data
ED, emergency department

practice, patients may instead be treated at a hospital. The impact is indirect, a reflection of the access or effectiveness of the ambulatory setting or both (Sarmento, 2020).

The Centers for Medicare and Medicaid Services (CMS) uses ACSCs to measure opportunities to improve quality, as evidenced by Table 4.2. CMS tracks both ambulatory care sensitive hospitalizations and emergency department (ED) visits. Because the data offer a reflection of the quality of an ambulatory practice, leaders may consider working with a hospital or health system partner, the government, an insurance company, or another stakeholder, to gather, monitor, and evaluate data about ACSCs. If patients can access ambulatory care and be effectively managed in an ambulatory practice, high-cost, unnecessary hospitalizations can be avoided. As such, these data are increasingly becoming a central focus of healthcare.

Quality Reporting

As the focus on quality has increased, the largest purchasers of healthcare in the United States—federal and state governments, as well as insurance companies—have implemented programs involving quality reporting. For example, the federal government launched a series of value-based payment programs designed, according to the CMS, to "reward health care providers with incentive payments for the quality of care they give to people with Medicare." For the federal government's programs, quality is measured in ambulatory practices in a multitude of ways. The Quality Payment Program (QPP) measures more than 200 quality metrics each year; providers can choose from quality measures based on efficiency, outcomes, patient engagement experience, patient-recorded outcome (PRO), process, and structure. Table 4.3 displays a sample of the QPP's quality measures, which are

TABLE 4.3 Select Measures in the Government's Quality Payment Program

QUALITY MEASURE	DESCRIPTION
ADVANCE CARE PLAN	Percentage of patients aged 65 years and older who have an advance care plan or surrogate decision-maker documented in the medical record or documentation in the medical record that an advance care plan was discussed but the patient did not wish or was not able to name a surrogate decision-maker or provide an advance care plan
APPROPRIATE TESTING FOR PHARYNGITIS	The percentage of episodes for patients three years and older with a diagnosis of pharyngitis that resulted in an antibiotic dispensing event and a group A streptococcus (strep) test
BREAST CANCER SCREENING	Percentage of women 50–74 years of age who had a mammogram to screen for breast cancer in the 27 months prior to the end of the measurement period
CERVICAL CANCER SCREENING	Percentage of women 21–64 years of age who were screened for cervical cancer using either of the following criteria: women age 21–64 who had cervical cytology performed within the last three years or women age 30–64 who had cervical human papillomavirus (HPV) testing performed within the last five years
CLOSING THE REFERRAL LOOP: RECEIPT OF SPECIALIST REPORT	Percentage of patients with referrals, regardless of age, for which the referring provider receives a report from the provider to whom the patient was referred
COLORECTAL CANCER SCREENING	Percentage of patients 50–75 years of age who had appropriate screening for colorectal cancer
CONTROLLING HIGH BLOOD PRESSURE	Percentage of patients 18–85 years of age who had a diagnosis of hypertension overlapping the measurement period and whose most recent blood pressure was adequately controlled (<140/90 mmHg) during the measurement period
DOCUMENTATION OF CURRENT MEDICATIONS IN THE MEDICAL RECORD	Percentage of visits for patients aged 18 years and older for which the eligible professional or eligible clinician attests to documenting a list of current medications using all immediate resources available on the date of the encounter
FALLS: SCREENING FOR FUTURE FALL RISK	Percentage of patients 65 years of age and older who were screened for future fall risk during the measurement period
FUNCTIONAL OUTCOME ASSESSMENT	Percentage of visits for patients aged 18 years and older with documentation of a current functional outcome assessment using a standardized functional outcome assessment tool on the date of the encounter *and* documentation of a care plan based on identified functional outcome deficiencies on the date of the identified deficiencies
IMMUNIZATIONS FOR ADOLESCENTS	The percentage of adolescents 13 years of age who had one dose of meningococcal vaccine (serogroups A, C, W, Y) and one tetanus, diphtheria toxoids and acellular pertussis (Tdap) vaccine and have completed the HPV vaccine series by their 13th birthday

(continued)

TABLE 4.3 Select Measures in the Government's Quality Payment Program (*Continued*)

QUALITY MEASURE	DESCRIPTION
MEDICATION MANAGEMENT FOR PEOPLE WITH ASTHMA	The percentage of patients 5–64 years of age during the performance period who were identified as having persistent asthma and were dispensed appropriate medications that they remained on for at least 75% of their treatment period
PNEUMOCOCCAL VACCINATION STATUS FOR OLDER ADULTS	Percentage of patients 65 years of age and older who have ever received a pneumococcal vaccine
PREVENTIVE CARE AND SCREENING: BODY MASS INDEX (BMI) SCREENING AND FOLLOW-UP PLAN	Percentage of patients aged 18 years and older with a BMI documented during the current encounter or within the previous 12 months AND who had a follow-up plan documented if most recent BMI was outside of normal parameters
SCREENING FOR OSTEOPOROSIS FOR WOMEN AGED 65–85 YEARS OF AGE	Percentage of female patients aged 65–85 years of age who have had a central dual-energy X-ray absorptiometry to check for osteoporosis

SOURCE: Quality Payment Program. (n.d.). 2021 quality measures. *Traditional MIPS*. https://qpp.cms.gov/mips/explore-measures?tab=qualityMeasures&py=2021

reported annually. The QPP, aimed at Medicare-participating providers, is one of myriad reporting opportunities for ambulatory practices. Read about the experience of a physician leader engaged in quality reporting in the sidebar "Quality Measurement." Enhanced technology is expanding opportunities to track and report metrics. Reporting of quality metrics is expected to increase in the future as healthcare purchasers (insurance companies), as well as consumers (patients), become more knowledgeable about using the data to assess outcomes of care.

The capacity of the ambulatory practice to establish goals for quality, monitor performance against those goals and continually improve performance along the identified quality dimensions provides the foundation for delivering quality care.

SAFETY

In 1999, the IOM released its landmark report, developed by the IOM Committee on Quality Health Care in America, called *To Err is Human: Building a Safer Health System*. One of the report's key findings was that an estimated 44,000 to 98,000 patient deaths occur per year in hospitals because of medical errors (IOM Committee on Quality of Health Care in America, 2000). This report brought to light the fact that the healthcare industry "could not address the overall quality of care without first addressing a key, but almost unrecognized component of quality; which was patient safety" (Donaldson, 2008).

QUALITY MEASUREMENT: THE COMPLEXITIES OF AN AMBULATORY PRACTICE

Manoj Jain, MD, MPH

Adjunct Professor

Department of Health Policy and Management

Rollins School of Public Health

Emory University

Atlanta, Georgia

When I served as the medical director for Tennessee's Quality Improvement Organization, the CMS piloted a quality improvement process for heart failure management in the outpatient setting in the early 1990s. I was eager, excited, and confident as I had successfully helped hospitals improve heart failure quality measures in the inpatient setting. Our initiative involved tracking outpatient measures (Butler et al., 2003), such as an echocardiogram report in the patient's chart and the prescription for an angiotensin-converting enzyme inhibitor or an angiotensin II receptor blocker for left ventricular systolic dysfunction. My enthusiasm was soon quelled as I learned that tracking and monitoring quality in the ambulatory setting is quite different than inpatient quality measurement.

After months of effort, we were able to recruit only a handful of practices for the pilot. The physicians had little or no incentives to collaborate for many reasons. First, there was inherent reticence simply based on the request for information. Why would an ambulatory practice engage with a government contractor to conduct a chart review to determine if an echocardiogram was performed or a cardiac prescription was given? Second, we encountered trepidation about the consequences for not performing according to the standard measures. Even for the small number of practices that agreed to participate, the physicians asked for reassurance that our organization would not "ding" them for poor performance. Third, the process itself was a time-intensive task. Trying to locate the echocardiogram report and abstracting medication data was a complicated, demanding responsibility, which added to the practice's overhead expense. Fourth, the practice's staff—already overstretched—often refused to spend time in an activity that did not involve direct patient care. Finally, the variability among one practice to another as to the documentation of the required data added to the complexity of the quality measurement process. All these factors stood in stark contrast to similar work in the hospital setting.

The end result was even more disconcerting than the measurement activity. When the analysis was finalized and the results showed poor performance, most physicians blamed the process. For example, they claimed that the echocardiogram was performed and the medications were given; however, the actions were not documented (or not reported in the "right" place to be measured). At the end of the pilot, everyone was pointing fingers—and no one was owning the opportunity to improve quality.

Times have changed. The CMS has altered its strategies to engage physicians, including my own practice. Each year, the administrator of my practice electronically tallies and submits to the federal government the details about the influenza vaccines we give to patients as a component of our participation in the government's QPP. As a physician, I make sure that our practice submits the data in an accurate and timely manner each year; otherwise, we incur a financial penalty. Aligning payment with quality made a critical difference in having practitioners accept and comply with quality improvement processes in the ambulatory setting. And, as important, electronic record keeping reduced the onerous burden associated with manually finding and reporting data.

Yet quality measurement and improvement in the ambulatory setting is not where it needs to be. To most doctors, including myself, quality measures are a checkbox, tasks I must perform to obtain my earned payment—or, better said, achieve the maximum possible payment available to me. These efforts do not reflect a checklist that is embraced by me or one that is embedded in my practice.

For quality improvement to be valued in the ambulatory setting, it needs to reflect a well-organized, team-based approach. Efforts must engage key stakeholders including the patient, as well as the care team (e.g., a health navigator, a nurse, and me).

Once ambulatory care reaches this ideal level of organized delivery, there will be integration and coordination. This will soon happen, but it will take time and effort. As a quality improvement advocate, I am thankful that the old days of pleading with doctors to participate in quality reporting efforts are gone but I look forward to the day when quality is hardwired into the day-to-day care provided in an ambulatory practice.

The report highlighted the growing complexity of the healthcare delivery system, including recognition of the burgeoning sector that is ambulatory care. The intricacy of the healthcare industry was compared to nuclear power plants, commercial aviation, and even bungee-jumping, all of which were viewed to be less risky than healthcare. The complicated environment was and continues to be extremely dependent on humans. Among the more notable recommendations was the need to address and improve the systems of care to reduce preventable medical errors. This recommendation stands in stark contrast to the historical approach to dealing with errors in medical care as caused by incompetent individuals. People were punished, but the processes and systems that gave rise to the errors remained. The report suggested a new approach that would require an organizational commitment to preventing, recognizing, and mitigating harm from human error.

As a result of the IOM report, patient safety was viewed as an integral, yet distinct, aspect of quality. Healthcare organizations, thus, began to apply the concepts of the Donabedian Model—structure, process, and outcome—to systematically assess errors to determine their cause or causes and then to redesign the care process to

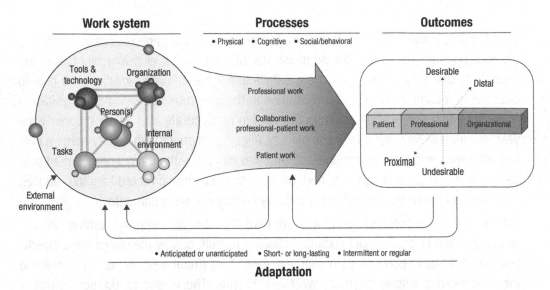

FIGURE 4.2 Systems engineering initiative for patient safety 2.0 model.

SOURCE: Holden, R. J., Carayon, P., Gurses, A. P., Hoonakker, P., Hundt, A. S., Ozok, A. A., & Rivera-Rodriguez, A. J. (2013). SEIPS 2.0: A human factors framework for studying and improving the work of healthcare professionals and patients. *Ergonomics, 56*(11), 1669–1686. https://doi.org/10.1080/00140139.2013.838643

remove the source(s) of the error, prevent the error from being repeated, and detect errors and mitigate harm for those that do occur. (Figure 4.2 presents the Systems Engineering Initiative for Patient Safety [SEIPS] 2.0 Model, which evolved from the Donabedian Model.) Patient safety models such as SEIPS 2.0 can be applied to evaluate and improve patient safety in an ambulatory practice.

Researcher James Reason (1997) furthered safety efforts through promulgating an approach that distinguishes between active failures and latent conditions. Human errors, Reason surmised, can be conceptualized like icebergs. Active failures are the observable elements of an error like the visible tip of the iceberg; however, there are also latent conditions that give way to safety problems (Reason, 1997). The active failure is the point at which the error occurred (e.g., the wrong medication is given). The person involved in the error (e.g., the nurse giving the wrong medication) is viewed as the cause of the problem.

Active errors only tell part of the story. The steps leading up to the active failure are the latent conditions. Like an iceberg, it is what lies under the surface that is often most dangerous and telling. Take the example of the nurse who gives the wrong medication to a patient. This is an example of an active failure, resulting in the possibility of a sentinel event that may cause harm to a patient. Giving the wrong medication is the endpoint of a potentially lengthy and complicated series of steps—the latent conditions—involving more than just the act of the nurse administering the wrong medication.

Latent conditions linger below the surface in the processes, systems, technology, and other people involved in the situation. Latent conditions may be attributable to inadequate staffing or other working conditions, communication failures, poor design, gaps in supervision, multiple uncoordinated hand-offs, or other process deficiencies, to name a few. Often unrecognized, the latent conditions contribute to the active failure that is ultimately observed.

The IOM's (2000) "*To Err is Human*" report suggests that focusing efforts on the actual mistake (e.g., retraining, counseling, or firing the nurse) will not likely result in a reduction of errors. Rather, the ambulatory practice in which this error occurred should systematically review the entire medication administration process, from its origin to the point at which the nurse administers the medication to the patient. Reason (1997) highlights this concept, stating that "we cannot change the human condition, but we can change the conditions under which people work" (Reason, 1997)

The heterogeneity of the ambulatory environment contributes to challenges regarding safety—and the research focused on improving it. Safety concerns in ambulatory practices are likely to be underreported (Kumar & Nash, 2021). Patient safety issues in the ambulatory setting may involve patient misidentification, missed, or delayed diagnoses (including the failure to follow-up on abnormal test results), untimeliness of proper treatment or preventive services, medication errors and adverse drug events, falls, and ineffective communication and information flow (ECRI Institute Patient Safety Organization, 2019; Sharma et al., 2021; Webster et al., 2008).

The sources of such errors vary as widely as the setting in which it takes place. Causal elements can be grouped into human factors and technical factors. Human factors may result from cognitive errors and the decision-making process, such as "failures in perception, failed heuristics, and decision-making biases" (Webster et al., 2008). Technical factors include lack of access to current technology, following out-of-date standards, a lack of appropriately trained staff, or relying on systems and processes that are manual in nature and error-prone. Factors contributing to quality and safety concerns in the ambulatory setting can be as mundane as failing to scan and properly index a patient's test result, relying on a patient's memory, or having a vacancy in a key staff position.

In efforts to align patient safety across a variety of healthcare settings, TJC established the National Patient Safety Goals in 2002, which continues to be updated annually in close collaboration with a panel of patient safety experts (TJC, 2021). These goals are established for a variety of healthcare settings, including ambulatory practices. Table 4.4 describes the 2021 National Patient Safety Goals specific to the ambulatory setting.

Every aspect of an ambulatory practice holds the opportunity to contribute or detract from the safety of care delivered to patients. Each appointment scheduled, each lab specimen collected, each message taken, each referral delivered, each health record documented, and many more processes contribute to a safe environment. Regardless of setting, safely delivering care is crucial in a well-managed ambulatory practice.

TABLE 4.4 National Patient Safety Goals for the Ambulatory Health Care Program

GOAL	RECOMMENDED ACTION
IMPROVE THE ACCURACY OF PATIENT IDENTIFICATION	• Use at least two patient identifiers when providing care, treatment, or services.
IMPROVE THE SAFETY OF USING MEDICATIONS	• Label all medications, medication containers, and other solutions on and off the sterile field in perioperative and other procedural settings. • Reduce the likelihood of patient harm associated with the use of anticoagulant therapy. • Maintain and communicate accurate patient medication information.
REDUCE THE RISK OF HEALTHCARE-ASSOCIATED INFECTIONS	• Comply with either the current Centers for Disease Control and Prevention hand hygiene guidelines and/or the current World Health Organization hand hygiene guidelines. • Create a preprocedure verification process. • Mark the procedure site. • A time-out is performed before the procedure.

SOURCE: The Joint Commission. (2020). *National patient safety goals effective January 2021 for the Ambulatory Health Care Program.* https://www.jointcommission.org/standards/national-patient-safety-goals/ambulatory-health-care-national-patient-safety-goals/

PATIENT EXPERIENCE

Quality, like beauty, is in the eye of the beholder. Although quality metrics in healthcare are most often focused on the structure, process, and outcome of the care rendered to a patient, the patient may have a different view of these elements. Patients—the consumers of care—may define quality based on their experience. This concept is so fundamental to a well-managed ambulatory practice that it justifies a distinct well of knowledge and resources.

In his teachings about quality, Donabedian (1992) acknowledged the role of the patient: "It is their [patients'] expectations that should set the standard for what is accessible, convenient, comfortable, or timely." He professed: "the quality of technical care is defined not by what is done, but by what is accomplished…technical care not congruent with patient preferences has failed in quality."

In formulating the framework for quality, Donabedian identified the fundamental role of the consumer; however, it was well into the 21st century before stakeholders determined how to integrate the pursuit and measurement of the patient experience in the ambulatory setting.

Consumerism

Unlike many other service industries, healthcare was not originally constructed with a focus on the preferences of the consumer. Although the goal has always been to deliver quality care, the means to achieve it—the structure, process, and outcome—were historically designed around the provider's needs and preferences. In many healthcare settings, the consumer—the patient—is an inactive participant. Consider, for example, a patient in the intensive care unit (ICU) in the hospital. They are likely prone in a bed, connected to machines, and immobile for much of the stay. In the ambulatory setting, however, patients are alert, engaged, and aware of all activities. The evaluation of experience commences before medical care is even provided. Patients gauge their experience on a culmination of moments of truth that occur over an encounter that begins before the physician enters the exam room Patient experience expert Susan Keane Baker (2009) defines *moments of truth* as "the moment your patient decides if you are what you say you are."

Despite Donabedian's professions about the role of the patient in the 1990s, it took nearly two decades for stakeholders to embrace patient experience as a priority in quality. Authors Don Berwick, MD; Thomas Nolan; and John Whittington propelled the concept of experience as a focus of attention with the *Triple Aim*. The Triple Aim featured the "simultaneous pursuit of . . . improving the experience of care, improving the health of populations, and reducing the per capita costs of health care" (Berwick, 2009). Figure 4.3 displays the framework of the Triple Aim. In the Triple Aim, patient experience refers to both improving the quality of care as well as the patient's satisfaction with the care delivery process, representing an evolution in the definition of quality in healthcare.

With experience gaining prominence, the federal government began using the Hospital Consumer Assessment of Healthcare Providers and Systems (HCAHPS) survey to impact hospital reimbursement in 2007 (CMS, 2021). Until this point,

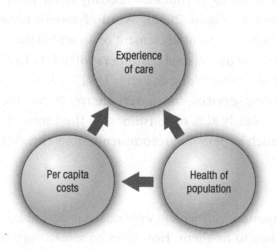

FIGURE 4.3 The Triple Aim.

SOURCE: Adapted from Berwick, D. M. (2009, May 19). What 'patient-centered' should mean: Confessions of an extremist. *Health Affairs, 28*(3/4), w555–w565. https://doi.org/10.1377/hlthaff.28.4.w555; Institute for Healthcare Improvement. (n.d.). *The IHI Triple Aim*. http://www.ihi.org/Engage/Initiatives/TripleAim/Pages/default.aspx

customer service was considered by many healthcare organizations as nice but not necessary. The CMS mandated that hospitals publicly report patient perceptions through HCAHPS surveys. The patient finally had a voice in a quality metric that impacted revenue.

The CMS expanded the standardized survey approach to include multiple ambulatory points of care: the CAHPS Clinician and Group Survey, the CAHPS Outpatient and Ambulatory Surgery Survey, and CAHPS Home Health Care Survey (AHRQ, 2019). Transparency in reporting has given consumers a standardized approach to comparing multiple providers and services, placing more control in consumers' hands.

Expectations

Today's consumers expect their healthcare providers to be as focused on customer service as any other service industry including, but not limited to, restaurants, hotels, spas, and theme parks. They want convenience, access, efficiency, transparency, state-of-the-art technology, and the latest, evidenced-based medical treatments—all delivered with the utmost respect, courtesy, and empathy.

Consumer demand is shaping healthcare delivery now more than ever. Consider the rapid emergence of walk-in clinics where patients can go when they choose to get care, not when an appointment is available. These clinics are available in retail stores, not just traditional medical office buildings. Patients today can simply scroll to an app on their phone to access care.

Meeting patients' expectations is a compelling business proposition. Research demonstrates that it is five to 25 times more costly to attract a new customer than to retain an existing one (Gallo, 2014). Word-of-mouth recommendations have been and continue to be an essential element of an ambulatory practice's success.

Research indicates that dissatisfied customers will tell 11 to 25 people about their experience (Hart et al., 1990; Wong & Perry, 1991). Today, with social media and dedicated online review services, consumers are free to rate their doctors and post their reviews online. Nearly 80% of consumers in the United States report trusting online reviews as much as personal recommendations (BrightLocal, 2020).

Design

Recognizing the importance of patient experience is desirable, but it is far easier to identify problems than to fix them. How does an ambulatory practice improve the patient experience?

The interaction with a product or service determines the consumer's overall impression and relationship with it. User experience has been studied and applied in numerous industries ranging from banking to theme parks, website design, and retail. Through an iterative process involving inspiration, ideation, and implementation, design thinking allows the provider to empathize with the consumer to create the most positive experience at each touch point (Brown, 2008; Rowe, 1987). Therefore, for healthcare operations to be truly patient-centered, the experience must be designed with patient input and focused on patients' preferences.

Berwick, former leader of the CMS and the Institute for Healthcare Improvement, revealed: "'Patient-centeredness' is a dimension of health care quality in its own right, not just because of its connection with other desired aims, like safety and effectiveness. Its proper incorporation into new health care designs will involve some radical, unfamiliar, and disruptive shifts in control and power, out of the hands of those who give care and into the hands of those who receive it." (Berwick, 2009).

The expectations of consumers have had a major impact on healthcare design, including technology, processes, and the environment. Take scheduling appointments, for example. Traditionally, appointments were made by calling the ambulatory practice during office hours, usually 8:00 a.m. to 5:00 p.m. A person at the practice answers the phone and speaks with the caller, trying to understand the caller's symptom or complaint(s). Once the reason for the visit is understood, the scheduler and the caller then attempt to find a mutually agreeable appointment. For some practices, this is only after a patient submits medical records for review and receives confirmation that an appointment can be made.

From the consumer's perspective, this traditional approach is fraught with a multitude of issues:

1. The consumer may not have or understand how to access to their medical records or be able to retrieve them in a timely manner, delaying the assessment phase. Importantly, there is no reimbursement for this time or effort—payment is only made when the patient is seen, not evaluated as to whether to be seen.

2. The consumer does not understand the reason for the assessment of records, if applicable; for example, what are the criteria to be selected for an appointment?

3. The consumer may be working and unable to make a call—particularly about a private matter like a medical appointment—during the traditional office hours.

4. The scheduler on the phone must search for openings before offering them to the caller.

5. The caller must check their schedule and accept or reject an offer of an appointment which can result in multiple back-and-forth attempts.

6. Appointments are often given weeks in advance, which may result in rescheduling if the caller's or provider's schedule changes or if the caller's symptoms escalate.

7. The scheduler is often interrupted by patients, providers, and other calls that further delay the resolution of the scheduling call.

Consumers want control over their time. They expect efficiency and convenience with access to scheduling on their terms. In thinking about the design of scheduling workflow considering these patient expectations, ambulatory practices have responded with the following:

1. Expansion of hours of operation for inbound calls

2. Reduction or elimination of pre-appointment medical records review processes

3. Addition of outbound communication processes, proactively initiated when a referral, order, or recommendation for preventive care is made (e.g., the practice calls or texts the patient about an appointment that was ordered or recommended)

4. Deployment of an omni-channel communication strategy, streamlining voice, text, chat, and secure electronic messaging

5. Execution of online scheduling platforms to allow patients to self-service their appointments; consumers can search for, and schedule, an appointment when it is convenient for them

In addition to advantaging the patient, there are benefits to the practice. These strategies may reduce practice costs, improve show rates, boost staff morale, and foster patient retention.

Design thinking has revolutionized the patient experience. **Journey mapping** is often the first step in designing the ideal patient experience. Journey mapping is the process of visualizing the steps a patient has from the moment they identify a need for a clinical visit. The assessment continues through every step of the encounter, including the patient's experience after the visit. The post-visit process may include a referral, order, transfer of care, or another process outside of the practice. Even though the patient is being sent to another entity, the hand-offs of care are just as important as getting a new patient in the door. Journey mapping—an exploration of touch points through the patient's journey—involves the examination of patient emotions, needs, and expectations at each phase, with comparisons against the actual experience to find opportunities for improvement.

See Figure 4.4 for a framework for journey mapping in an ambulatory practice. Stakeholders can determine the various components that influence the patient's decision-making at each stage in the journey. Consistent with quality and safety, using the framework of structure, process, and outcomes can help identify opportunities for improvement. See the following sidebar for a deep dive into one aspect of structure—the design elements of the physical environment in an ambulatory

DEEP DIVE INTO THE PHYSICAL ENVIRONMENT

Donald Norman, a cognitive scientist and engineer who pioneered the concept of user-centered design, has brought forth several key concepts that bolster the design of systems, processes, and products to prevent human error. In his book *The Design of Everyday Things*, Norman (1988) discusses the following principles in user-centered design: (a) make things visible, including the interface and conceptual framework of the system or process, (b) simplify tasks to minimize memory, planning, and problem-solving, (c) use "affordances" (cues on how to operate a device or system), and (d) use "restraints" (features or functions that make it hard to do the wrong thing). These considerations have high relevance to healthcare processes and technologies today, which recognize the impact of human factors on process design and user experience to minimize error (Norman, 1988).

The physical environment is crucial to patient's perceptions of their experience. Although aesthetics is important in creating an impression, functionality is equally crucial to creating ease of use of the practice's facility. On the most basic level, one should consider the senses when designing the patient care environment.

Visual: Graphic appeal, lighting, and use of space have a significant influence on patient impressions. In addition to signs, consider visual cues that guide the patient toward a point. Colors or shapes may be used instead of numbers or names. Consider a multispecialty practice with women's health clinics for urologic gynecology, reproductive endocrinology, and maternal–fetal medicine. Wayfinding may be improved by using colors or shapes instead of these lengthy names. Maintaining a clean and clutter-free environment communicates professionalism and helps evoke trust.

Sound: Loud noise, including talking, phones ringing, doors banging, and other sounds, can create stress and a feeling of being confused and overwhelmed, which can raise a patient's stress level. Because confidentiality is vital in healthcare, it is essential to consider how voices carry and work to control privacy.

Smell: Patients are often sensitive to smell, especially when they are not feeling well. Maintaining a clean environment diminishes odors in the building. Staff play a part and should be reminded to avoid food odors and strong perfumes.

The physical environment offers the opportunity for an ambulatory practice to improve the patient experience.

practice. Take a further step into the crucial elements of an exam room in Figure 4.5 and Exhibit 4.2 and the accompanying materials by learning the key design principles to consider for the exam rooms in a well-managed ambulatory practice.

A great patient experience in an ambulatory practice is a business imperative as it encourages loyalty and builds positive word of mouth. Creating a consistently

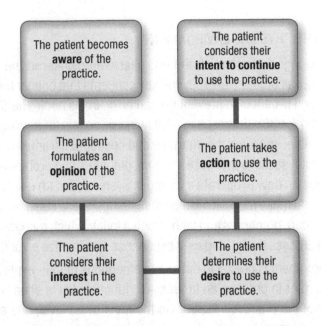

FIGURE 4.4 Stages of journey map.

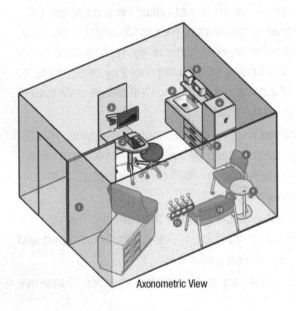

Axonometric View

1. Reverse door swing to hide exam table when door is ajar
2. Height-adjustable, mobile table for keyboard use with monitor and/or laptop to optimize sightlines between clinician and patient/family
3. Monitor on adjustable arm to support virtual visit and in-person information sharing
4. Handwashing in the natural path/position of clinician
5. Rail or Shelf reduces clutter and avoids sink splash
6. Rotated shelving to mitigate patient/family exposure to clinical tools and reduce clutter.
7. Integral waste receptacle off the floor for ease of cleaning
8. Patient/family seating oriented to face the door and easily view the clinician/monitor. Chairs are sturdy but moveable.
9. Patient/family worksurface within easy reach for note taking, devices
10. Wider seat to accommodate people of size and/or parent and child, located adjacent to the exam table for support
11. Accommodate belongings near the patient/family

FIGURE 4.5 Key considerations of exam room design.

SOURCE: Michelle Ossmann and Jolene DeJong (Herman Miller Healthcare).

positive patient experience occurs by design, not by chance. It begins by under-standing the patient's journey. Setting standards ensures consistency from one person or department to the next. Strong leadership is essential to the patient

EXHIBIT 4.2 CHECKLIST FOR EXAM ROOM DESIGN CONSIDERATIONS

Safety

Patient and Family

☐ Infection control
  ☐ Cleanability - technology and surfaces EPA wipeable; easy-to-clean design
  ☐ Handwashing - visible; easy access to sink and waterless options
☐ Injury prevention - rounded corners and edges; chairs with arms; adjustable height as appropriate
  ☐ Information sharing - video and face-to-face; main same-level site lines while using screens

Clinician

☐ Infection control
  ☐ Cleanability - technology and surfaces EPA wipeable; easy-to-clean design
  ☐ Handwashing - visible; easy access to sink and waterless options
  ☐ Waste handling - easy access to trash and linen
☐ Injury prevention
  ☐ Ergonomics - height adjustable exam surface and documentation set-up
  ☐ Aggressive patients - orientation of entry and exit
  ☐ Needlesticks and other injuries - sharps containers location

Experience

Patient and Family

☐ Information sharing
  ☐ Circle of trust - same-level site lines, accomodation of patient's advocates
  ☐ Information sharing - video and face-to-face; surfaces on which to write and place items
  ☐ Acoustic and visual privacy - exam table hidden when door ajar; room sound ratings
☐ Hosting
  ☐ Belongings - place to hang clothes, bags, purses, etc., off of the floor
  ☐ Seating - comfortable; accounting for persons of various body types

Clinician

☐ Information sharing
  ☐ Circle of trust - same-level site lines, accomodation of patient's advocates
  ☐ Information sharing - video and face-to-face; surfaces on which to write and place items
☐ Efficiency
  ☐ EHR system - access and orientation to share screens with patient and family as appropriate
  ☐ Exam table - location and function supportive of efficent interactions
  ☐ Supplies - oft-used supplies at hand; inactive supplies well-organized
  ☐ Support staff - accommodation of care team with seating and documentation

SOURCE: Michelle Ossmann and Jolene DeJong (Herman Miller Healthcare).

experience; like any aspect of quality in an ambulatory practice, it does not represent a singular event.

IMPROVEMENT STRATEGIES

To promote improvements in quality, safety, and patient experience, ambulatory practices require a clear strategy, competent clinical and administrative leadership, and an evidence-informed approach. The goal for ambulatory leadership is to assure that stakeholders are focused on improving the processes of care to eliminate or reduce

THE IDEAL EXAM ROOM FOR A WELL-MANAGED AMBULATORY PRACTICE

Michelle Ossmann, PhD, MSN, Assoc. AIA

Director of Knowledge and Innovation

Herman Miller Healthcare

Zeeland, Michigan

The design of an ambulatory practice is a critical determinant in the delivery of safe, quality care. The physical layout of an exam room, the location of care delivery in the ambulatory setting, can promote a positive experience for patients and families while providing an efficient and effective work setting for clinicians and other team members. Successful outcomes require support for the full care team—patients, families, clinicians, and staff. To accomplish the practice's goals for safety, quality, and experience, well-managed ambulatory practices should aim to incorporate five key design principles in constructing an exam room:

Safety—Infection control and cleanability are the baseline requirement and cannot be compromised as design elements. Prioritizing easy handwashing upon entry and during the clinical encounter as necessary is a key design consideration. Careful integration of common supplies, such as sharps containment, paper towels, gloves, and a trash receptacle, supports rigid cleanliness and safety protocols. Accidental injury is mitigated with rounded corners and edges on surfaces and sturdy patient and family seating with arms.

Patient privacy—Maintaining confidentiality and bodily privacy is a hallmark of experience, and the exam room is a key factor in supporting the practice's effort to deliver it. Focusing on "hiding" the exam table (or chair) when the door is ajar is a vital design element, as is attention to the acoustic integrity of the room. Adjacent workspaces also affect actual and perceived confidentiality and should be designed to support informational privacy and the communication needs of the care team.

Communication—Be mindful of the nature of the information being exchanged by creating spaces that advocate trust. This "circle of trust" can be considered as a convex polygon where everyone is on the same level of visibility and transparency, including digital and analog information displays. Information is its own actor and requires careful attention. Exam rooms are the places where relationships are built whether it is a routine visit, a physical exam, or a consultation. By understanding the clinicians' or team members' work in the context of the circle of trust, defined and tacit communication tools and technology can be integrated into the design. Considerations may include accommodating telepresence such that a dual monitor can be used to engage with a remote participant or review data from the patient's electronic health record with the patient and family.

Family presence—A patient's health is often a shared experience with loved ones, caregivers, and others who are supporting the patient's journey. The exam room should provide space to host and include the patient's advocate; design elements include the storage of belongings, benches, cushion top laterals, extra side chairs, and the ability for the patient's supporters to physically reside near the patient in the exam room.

Operational flexibility—An exam room must be designed with an eye to efficiency for the clinician, with adaptability as the key element to avoid design obsolescence. The facility may accommodate a place for additional team members, such as a navigator, in the exam room and perhaps a secondary mobile surface on which to write or use a technology device. Furthermore, the exam room should allow for storage, furnishing, and technology organization to adapt the room to changing functions, specialties, or exam types. Tools and supplies should be arranged for easy, flexible access, and include active supplies on display in shelves or open cubbies, as well as inactive supplies arranged in drawers or rails.

Figure 4.5 displays key considerations of exam room design. Use the accompanying checklist in Exhibit 4.2 as you evaluate the design elements for an ambulatory practice. In constructing exam rooms for the well-managed ambulatory practice, however, design cannot be considered in a vacuum. Process and policy need to work in concert with the environment.

clinical and administrative errors, which, in turn, have been shown to enhance patient outcomes, facilitate the safe provision of care, and enhance the patient experience. To accomplish these goals, the well-managed ambulatory practice considers vision, data, team orientation, and sustainability in constructing the improvement strategies.

Vision

Developing the strategic vision to improve patient quality, safety, and experience requires committed leaders, clinicians, and personnel partnering to create the idea and understand the problems. Leaders must be willing to role model the desired behaviors to secure buy-in from all personnel. As part of the visioning process, it is important to share relevant and compelling stories related to quality, safety, and process deficiencies.

According to David Hutchens (2015), telling stories is one of the most powerful means that leaders have to influence, teach, and inspire. Storytelling allows for understanding ("I get it, I understand why this is important"), alignment ("I'm in, let's do this"), and action ("What can we do, now?"). Clear, concise, and honest communication is critical to all improvement efforts. Every attempt must be made to open channels of communication at all levels in an ambulatory practice. The goals for communicating effectively around quality, safety, and experience concerns are to eliminate the fear associated with surfacing concerns, promote team accountability for performance, provide accurate and timely feedback, engage all relevant stakeholders including patients, and build trust. It is also important that this vision is shared across all personnel. In the book *Managing the Risks of Organizational*

Accidents, author James Reason (1997) describes the concept of "just culture": "Just culture creates an atmosphere of trust in which people are encouraged to provide, and even rewarded for providing, essential safety-related information but in which they are clear about where the line must be drawn between acceptable and unacceptable behavior" (Reason, 1997).

Data

With a clear vision or purpose established, the goal is to review existing practice metrics to assess performance along the dimensions measured. To the extent there are existing data, a thorough evaluation of these data is necessary. There are several questions to consider. Are these data reliable and valid? Can the data be presented and explained to stakeholders? Do stakeholders believe the numbers? Are there targets or benchmarks established for the measures? If benchmarks are used, are the benchmarks selected comparable (e.g., same specialty, practice type, etc.)? How often are these reported and with whom are they shared? Finally, do personnel, including providers, understand how the measures relate to the desired outcomes, and how they may impact performance?

Improvement efforts may be boosted by accessing externally developed and tested standards and data. Key data sources include, but are not limited to, the Agency for Healthcare Research and Quality (AHRQ), the Consumer Assessment of Healthcare Providers and Systems (CAHPS) Ambulatory Care Improvement Guide and the National Healthcare Quality and Disparities Report (Ambulatory), the National Quality Forum (NQF), National Committee for Quality Assurance (NCQA), and The Joint Commission (TJC).

Many practices have their own quality, safety, and experience measures; they may be extracted or adapted from a professional association or specialty society. Finally, there may be comparable data based on a payer's program, such as the CMS's Ambulatory Surgical Center Quality Reporting Program. The data may also be a function of participation in an accountable care organization, clinically integrated network, or other entity in which the practice is involved. Well-managed practices embrace the opportunity to compare data and improve.

The goal in this step is to collect meaningful performance data, establish targets for expected performance, assess performance against those targets over time, prioritize areas requiring attention, and then take action.

Team

Once priority areas are established, the leadership of the practice—or the team to which they have delegated the responsibility to lead the improvement efforts—must create a team-based approach to addressing the areas identified. The complexity of an ambulatory practice necessitates engaging multiple stakeholders; with a few exceptions, improvement requires multiple people and processes.

Improvement efforts involve several steps. First, assemble a team of subject-matter experts in the area to be addressed. In many instances, this may be internal staff. In some cases, it may be necessary to reach out for assistance if internal expertise is lacking or to bolster new perspectives. After assembling the team, provide the team with the existing data. Allow the team to review the data, discuss performance, and, together with the leaders of the improvement efforts, establish clear targets and timelines for improvement. With the team, targets, and timelines established, it is necessary to discuss the approach that will be used to improve performance. This is where the leadership can provide resources (e.g., support, protected time to work on the issue, etc.) and performance improvement tools to guide the effort.

Using evidence-based improvement concepts like Edwards Deming's PDSA model (The W. Edwards Deming Institute, 2021), Situation-Background-Assessment-Recommendation (SBAR) (IHI, 2021), and Team Strategies and Tools to Enhance Performance and Patient Safety (TeamSTEPPS) (AHRQ, 2021) can facilitate efforts. As demonstrated in Figure 4.6, TeamSTEPPS presents a framework of four teachable, learnable skills to optimize team performance. See https://www.youtube.com/watch?v=1JBJ7zBNCgY for an exercise that demonstrates key skills for the team environment. **Process improvement** tools like cause-and-effect diagrams, process flow diagrams, time and motion studies, and other data collection activities can further improvement efforts. This may require team training in these important concepts before embarking on the assigned improvement journey or introducing an outside resource to facilitate the use of the appropriate methods and tools.

Sustainability

In redesigning processes to improve quality, reduce errors, and enhance satisfaction with achieving desired outcomes, the leadership should focus on accountability, integrity, and monitoring—their AIM (Bittle & Charache, 2008). To promote sustainability in process improvement, leadership must assure that for each complete process (e.g., medication administration), as well as the sub-elements of processes (e.g., entering the medication order), there is clear accountability established. Another necessary element for sustainable improvement is integrity. Every process must be designed to produce the result desired. For example, failure to address and follow up on abnormal test results is a significant problem for some ambulatory practice settings. The process improvement team focused on assuring appropriate action is taken should design a formal process that oversees, reviews, and follows up on any abnormal results within an identified timeframe. A process designed from the outset to produce the desired result can be considered to have integrity—in other words, it can be counted on doing what it is supposed to do.

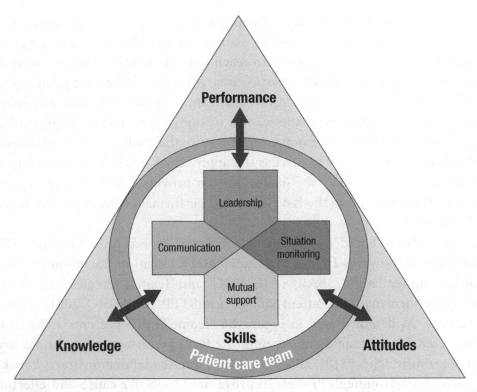

FIGURE 4.6 Team strategies and tools to enhance performance and patient safety (TeamSTEPPS).

SOURCE: Agency for Healthcare Research and Quality. (2021, February 20). **TeamSTEPPS**. https://www.ahrq.gov/teamstepps/index.html

To complete the creation of sustainable performance improvement, the leadership must assure appropriate metrics and monitoring systems are in place. The measures selected should be ones that have been shown to have a clear cause-and-effect relationship with the desired outcome. The measure type is also important, especially in the ambulatory setting, where there are typically high-volume events. For example, using absolute numbers or time to event units may be preferred for "never" events because the goal is zero, while using rates (e.g., percentage of total patients seen) may not adequately capture the event in question. A 1% error rate may not seem to some to require attention, but the interpretation depends heavily on the denominator. If there are more than a million patient encounters per annum in the ambulatory enterprise of a health system, that represents 1,000 errors each year.

Metrics are only useful if there is a monitoring system in place. The monitoring system should be designed based on the relative impact of an error resulting from a process deviation. The higher the potential for harm, the more frequent reporting is needed (e.g., daily monitoring). Establishing accountability for processes, especially critical events (i.e., events more likely to produce harm), assuring processes are designed with integrity to produce the desired results, and verifying appropriate metrics and monitoring are in place have been demonstrated to enhance the sustainability of performance improvement initiatives (Bittle & Charache, 2008).

CONCLUSION

A well-managed ambulatory practice ensures that evidence-based processes are in place to assure quality, safety, and patient experience are at the forefront of all activities. Leadership commitment, a clear and compelling vision, a structured, data-driven approach, aligned interest and incentives, and the application of proven tools and techniques are essential to the success of improving quality, safety, and patient experience.

DISCUSSION QUESTIONS

1. Why is defining, measuring, and assuring quality challenging in the ambulatory setting?

2. What role does accreditation play in assuring the quality and safety of medical care?

3. What are the differences between what is referred to as "quality of medical care" and "patient safety"?

4. You are a new ambulatory practice manager and asked to establish a quality and safety program. Describe important elements you would include. How might these differ from the inpatient setting?

5. Missed or delayed diagnosis is a top area of concern in the ambulatory setting. Explain why this poses a risk to patients. Why this is more likely to occur in an ambulatory setting?

6. What is "patient-centered care" and how does this concept relate to improving quality and the patient experience?

7. What is the concept of patient experience and why it is included as part of the Triple Aim?

8. What role does continuous improvement play and why is it an essential element to improving ambulatory quality, safety, and the patient experience?

9. Why is sustainability so important? What are some ways to assure sustainability in the quality program in an ambulatory practice?

10. Who are the key players in developing, implementing, and monitoring quality, safety, and the patient experience in the ambulatory care setting? Explain your reason for each.

REFERENCES

Agency for Healthcare Research and Quality. (2001, October). *Guide to prevention quality indicators: Hospital admission for ambulatory care sensitive conditions*. Agency for Healthcare Research and Quality. https://www.ahrq.gov/downloads/pub/ahrqqi/pqiguide.pdf

Agency for Healthcare Research and Quality. (2018, February). *Ambulatory care*. Agency for Healthcare Research and Quality. https://www.ahrq.gov/patient-safety/settings/ambulatory/tools.html

Agency for Healthcare Research and Quality. (2019, August). *CAHPS patient experience surveys and guidance*. https://www.ahrq.gov/cahps/surveys-guidance/index.html

Agency for Healthcare Research and Quality. (2021, February 20). *TeamSTEPPS*. Agency for Healthcare Research and Quality. https://www.ahrq.gov/teamstepps/index.html

Baker, S. K. (2009). *Managing patient expectations: The art of finding and keeping loyal patients*. Jossey-Bass.

Berman, P. (2000). Organization of ambulatory care provision: A critical determinant of health system performance in developing countries. *Bulletin of the World Health Organization, 78*(6), 791–802.

Berwick, D. M. (2009, May 19). What 'patient-centered' should mean: Confessions of an extremist. *Health Affairs, 28*(3/4), w555–w565. https://doi.org/10.1377/hlthaff.28.4.w555

Billings, J. Z. L. (1993). Impact of socioeconomic status on hospital use in New York City. *Health Affairs, 12*(1), 162–173. https://doi.org/10.1377/hlthaff.12.1.162

Bittle, M. J., & Charache, P. (2008). Taking "AIM" at lasting change: Self-sustaining improvement in patient identification. In T. J. Commission (Ed.), *Implementing and sustaining improvement in health care* (pp. 119–126). Joint Commission Resources.

BrightLocal. (2020). *Local consumer review survey 2020*. https://www.brightlocal.com/research/local-consumer-review-survey

Brown, T. (2008). Design thinking. *Harvard Business Review, 86*(6), 84–92.

Butler, J., Weingarten, J. P., Jr., Weddle, J. A., & Jain, M. K. (2003). Differences among hospitals in delivery of care for heart failure. *Journal for Healthcare Quality, 25*(3), 4–10, quiz 11, 39. https://doi.org/10.1111/j.1945-1474.2003.tb01052.x

Centers for Disease Control and Prevention. (2010). *National ambulatory medical care survey*. https://www.cdc.gov/nchs/data/ahcd/namcs_summary/2010_namcs_web_tables.pdf

Centers for Medicare and Medicaid Services. (2020). *CY 2021 Medicare hospital outpatient prospective payment system and ambulatory surgical center payment system final rule (CMS-1736-FC)*. https://www.cms.gov/newsroom/fact-sheets/cy-2021-medicare-hospital-outpatient-prospective-payment-system-and-ambulatory-surgical-center-0

Centers for Medicare and Medicaid Services. (2021). *CMS measures inventory tool. Hospitalization for ambulatory care sensitive*. https://cmit.cms.gov/CMIT_public/ReportMeasure?measureRevisionId=933

Dobson, J. L., & Jones, M. F. (2004, September/October). Making healthcare 'patient-centered': The centerpiece of quality improvement. *North Carolina Medical Journal, 65*(5), 295–297. https://doi.org/10.18043/ncm.65.5.295

Donabedian, A. (1992). Quality assurance in health care: Consumers' role. *Quality in Health Care, 1*, 247–251. https://www.ncbi.nlm.nih.gov/pmc/articles/PMC1055035/pdf/qualhc00004-0035.pdf

Donabedian, A. (2003). *An introduction to quality assurance in health care*. Oxford University Press.

Donabedian, A. (2005). Evaluating the quality of medical care. *The Milbank Quarterly, 83*(4), 691–729. https://doi.org/10.1111/j.1468-0009.2005.00397.x

Donaldson, M. S. (2008). An overview of to err is human: Re-emphasizing the message of patient safety. In H. Rg (Ed.), *Patient safety and quality: An evidence-based handbook for nurses* (Chapter 3). Agency for Healthcare Research and Quality. https://www.ncbi.nlm.nih.gov/books/NBK2673/

ECRI Institute Patient Safety Organization. (2019). *Safe ambulatory care. Strategies for patient safety & risk reduction.* https://assets.ecri.org/PDF/Deep-Dives/ECRI-PSO-DD-Ambulatory-Care-2019.pdf

Federal Aviation Administration. (2009). *Risk management handbook. FAA-H-8083-2.* https://www.faa.gov/regulations_policies/handbooks_manuals/aviation/media/risk_management_hb_change_1.pdf

Food and Drug Association. (2009). *Guidance for industry on patient-reported outcome measures: Use in medical product development to support labeling claims.*

Gallo, A. (2014). The value of keeping the right customers. *Harvard Business Review*, October 29.

Hart, W. L., Heskett, J. L., & Sasser, W. E., Jr. (1990). The profitable art of service recovery. *Harvard Business Review*, July–August, 148–156.

Hutchens, D. (2015). *Circle of the 9 muses: A storytelling field guide for innovators & meaning makers.* John Wiley & Sons.

Institute for Healthcare Improvement. (2021). *SBAR tool: Situation-background-assessment-recommendation.* http://www.ihi.org/resources/Pages/Tools/SBARToolkit.aspx

Institute of Medicine (US) Committee on Quality of Health Care in America. (2000). *To err is human: Building a safer health system.* National Academies Press.

Institute of Medicine (US) Committee to Design a Strategy for Quality Review and Assurance in Medicare. (1990). *Medicare: A strategy for quality assurance.* Edited by K. N. Lohr. National Academic Press.

Karnofsky, D. A., Abelmann, W. H., Craver, L. F., & Burchenal, J. H. (1948). The use of the nitrogen mustards in the palliative treatment of carcinoma—With particular reference to bronchogenic carcinoma. *Cancer, 1*(4), 634–656. https://doi.org/10.1002/1097-0142(194811)1:4[[634::AID-CNCR2820010410]]3.0.CO;2-L

Kumar, P. R., & Nash, D. B. (2021). Annotated bibliography: An update to "understanding ambulatory carepractices in the context of patient safety and quality improvement". *American Journal of Medical Quality, 36*(3), 185–196. https://doi.org/10.1177/1062860620938762

Lewis, N. (2014, October 17). *A primer on defining the triple aim.* Institute for Healthcare Improvement. http://www.ihi.org/communities/blogs/a-primer-on-defining-the-triple-aim

Neuhauser, D. (2002, March 1). Ernest Amory Codman MD. *Quality and Safety in Health Care, 11*, 104–105. https://doi.org/10.1136/qhc.11.1.104

Norman, D. (1988). *The design of everyday things.* Basic Books.

Preidecker, P. (2019, November/December). Putting TEM on your safety team. *FAA Safety Briefing* (pp. 8–11). https://www.faa.gov/news/safety_briefing/2019/media/NovDec2019.pdf

Reason, J. (1997). *Managing the risks of organizational accidents.* Ashgate Publishing.

Rowe, P. (1987). *Design thinking.* MIT Press.

Sarmento, J. R. (2020). Defining ambulatory care sensitive conditions for adults in Portugal. *BMC Health Services Research, 20*(1), 754. https://doi.org/10.1186/s12913-020-05620-9

Sharma, A. E., Yang, J., Rosario, J. B., Hoskote, M., Rivadeneira, N. A., Council, S. R., & Sarkar, U. (2021, January). What safety events are reported for ambulatory care? Analysis of incident reports from a patient safety organization. *The Joint Commission Journal on Quality and Patient Safety, 47*(1), 5–14. https://doi.org/10.1016/j.jcjq.2020.08.010

The Joint Commission. (2020). *The Joint Commission: Over a century of quality and safety.* https://www.jointcommission.org/about-us/facts-about-the-joint-commission/history-of-the-joint-commission/

The W. Edwards Deming Institute. (2021, February 20). *PDSA cycle.* The W. Edwards Deming Institute. https://deming.org/explore/pdsa/

Webster, J. S., King, H. B., Toomey, L. M., Salisbury, M. L., Powell, S. M., Craft, B., Baker, D. P., & Salas, E. (2008). Understanding quality and safety problems in the ambulatory environment: Seeking improvement with promising teamwork tools and strategies. In K. Henriksen (Ed.), *Advances in patient safety: New directions and alternative approaches* (Vol. 3: Performance and Tools). Agency for Healthcare Research and Quality. https://www.ncbi.nlm.nih.gov/books/NBK43683/

Wong, S. M., & Perry, C. (1991). Customer service strategies in financial retailing. *International Journal of Bank Marketing, 9*(3), 11–16.

OPERATIONS

LEARNING OBJECTIVES

1. Determine the stages of ambulatory operations
2. Understand the evolution and application of the electronic health record system in ambulatory practices
3. Recognize the emergence of **telemedicine** in ambulatory practice
4. Understand performance improvement opportunities in ambulatory practice

KEY TERMS

Registration	Standing Orders
Portal	Referral
Social Determinants of Health	Prior Authorization
Template	Huddle
Appointment Duration	Telemedicine
Self-Scheduling	Escalation
Waitlist	Care Transitions
Clinical Intake	Lean Production

INTRODUCTION

The patient's journey to care often commences in the ambulatory setting. Whether it is referred to as a "doctor's office," "outpatient clinic," or "medical practice," there are clinical and business workflows specific to the ambulatory setting. Alignment and integration of both clinical and business work functions throughout the ambulatory practice permit patients to receive optimal care and service, while ensuring the financial health of the practice.

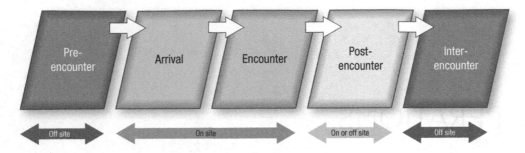

FIGURE 5.1 Stages of ambulatory practice operations.

PATIENT FLOW

In this chapter, we review and discuss the five stages of ambulatory operations: (1) pre-encounter, (2) arrival, (3) encounter, (4) post-encounter, and (5) inter-encounter, as depicted in Figure 5.1.

Stage 1: Pre-Encounter

As the name suggests, the pre-encounter stage takes place prior to the patient being seen. It involves two specific activities: (1) **registration** and (2) scheduling. Registration ensures the patient's demographic and insurance information are posted to the electronic health record (EHR) system so there is a formal record of the patient. Scheduling involves matching the patient's concerns or needs with the appropriate clinician, encounter duration, and timeliness to care. Collectively, these two activities are referred to as scheduling and registration; some have even dubbed these entwined processes as "schedgistration."

Registration and Scheduling

The patient contacts the ambulatory practice via phone, **portal**, or other communication mechanism; or utilizes an online, self-service system. Regardless of the mechanism, before the patient is appointed on the schedule, a registration process occurs. First and foremost, the patient is identified. The Joint Commission, which requires two identifiers for its accredited practices, defines a patient identifier as "information directly associated with an individual that reliably identifies the individual as the person for whom the service or treatment is intended" (TJC, 2020a). Acceptable identifiers, according to TJC, may be "the individual's name, an assigned identification number, telephone number, or other person-specific identifier" (TJC, 2020b). The identification process varies by ambulatory practice; however, the patient's name and date of birth are commonly used patient identifiers. Proper patient identification, applied in a consistent, systematic fashion, is crucial to the registration process. Accurate patient identification is the foundation of patient safety and financial health in an ambulatory practice.

After the patient is identified, the registration process continues with obtaining the patient's demographic and insurance information. This includes patient identifiers that have not yet been gathered such as date of birth, as well as the patient's phone number(s) and address.

Insurance information is collected by asking the patient the name of the insurance company or health plan and accompanying identification numbers. This segment of the process may be referred to as "financial clearance" because details are gathered to determine the party that is financially responsible for the services to be rendered to the patient. The information gathered from the patient at this stage may be brief, thereby the name, "mini-registration"—or it may be extensive. The ambulatory practice determines the details of the registration process.

Once registration information is obtained, the process of scheduling involves matching the patient with the appropriate appointment date, time, duration, and provider. This requires gleaning information from the patient about their health concerns or needs. For example, if the patient requests an annual physical examination, the appointment slot may be longer than the time reserved for a patient complaining of ear pain. Akin to registration, the process may be simple or detailed based on the type of ambulatory practice.

Although patient identification and clinical data are gathered by the conclusion of the registration and scheduling process, the flow of the transaction may differ among ambulatory practices. In some practices, the mini-registration occurs prior to scheduling the appointment. In these practices, basic details are first obtained from the patient, such as name, date of birth, and insurance type. Then, an inquiry is made about the patient's clinical concern. Next, an appointment slot is selected by the patient based on real-time availability. After the appointment date and time are secured, the balance of the registration takes place, such as obtaining full insurance identification (including group and plan numbers), emergency contact information, and **referral** source. Scheduling typically precedes the completion of the full registration because the patient is assured an appointment slot. If full registration comes first but no appointment is available, then the registration would have been futile. In some ambulatory settings, this process is bifurcated into two separate interactions with the patient: A mini-registration and scheduling transaction consume the initial touchpoint with the patient, followed by a second outbound communication to the patient to complete the full registration.

Increasingly, elements of the registration process are migrating to an online, self-service platform that allows asynchronous communication between the patient and the provider. Some ambulatory practices have transitioned all phone-based procedures to an online format; others have determined procedures that vary between new or established patients. For example, new patients, often defined as a patient who has not received services from a given practice in the past three years, may be directed to initiate communication through a phone-based interaction. In contrast, the entire registration process may be completed online for established patients. This may include collecting data regarding demographics and insurance and may extend beyond the registration process into assembling the patient's medical history. The process may also extend to the practice's site where a kiosk or tablet may be used to confirm key data elements related to the registration process in lieu of asking the patient to provide the information verbally. The use of advanced technologies to facilitate self-service registration come with several key benefits, such as labor cost savings for the practice, convenience for the patient, and data accuracy.

Once the registration and scheduling process is complete, significant work processes are typically conducted behind the scenes:

- **Data Verification.** Patient data gathered during the scheduling call may be verified internally. This includes the patient's address and insurance information, both of which can be manually or often electronically validated against databases. For example, the insurance coverage may be confirmed with the patient's insurance company; this process, typically performed electronically and without manual intervention, is referred to as the eligibility process. The process may stop here, or it may continue with a clinical review. This extent of the data verification process varies significantly by ambulatory practice, as it is dictated by the needs of the patient as well as the clinician. For example, the patient may be contacted to collect additional medical information; alternatively, this may be requested of all patients via electronic means. The clinical data may prompt a workflow in preparation for the patient's arrival, such as preordering a lab test, imaging study, any therapies, or other instructions.

- **Appointment Triage.** Attention may be given to the patient's clinical reason for appointment. This involves reviewing the patient's stated concern to determine whether the timing and duration of the appointment are appropriate, as well as whether the patient has been scheduled with the appropriate provider. This form of appointment triage is typically done after an appointment is booked; however, there are some practices that require these details to be reviewed before an appointment slot is confirmed.

- **Social Determinants of Health.** Recognizing the importance of social determinants of health and the implications on patient's needs, ambulatory practices may integrate questions during the pre-encounter process. This may guide the choice of clinician and/or time for the encounter; alternatively, information gleaned about social determinants of health may aid the clinician in providing more personalized care.

- **Escalation Protocols.** It is common for an **escalation** protocol to be followed based on certain clinical complaints expressed by the patient. This ensures that any emergent or acute patient concerns are addressed for proper follow-up during the standard process. As an example, if a patient complains of chest pain, that patient may be immediately triaged to speak with a nurse over the phone, instructed to hang up and call 911, or be directed to the nearest emergency department. In this manner, when a patient is describing his or her concerns during the scheduling process and certain clinical complaints are expressed, the personnel collecting these details can take immediate action to assist the patient.

- **Patient Outreach.** Once the patient is scheduled, a review of the schedule typically takes place prior to the visit date. Based on this review, the practice may reach out to the patient to conduct additional activities. The patient, for example, may be rescheduled to an earlier or later date based on the urgency of the patient's clinical condition. The patient's registration details may also alert personnel to converse with the patient regarding their insurance. As an example, the type of insurance may require the patient to obtain a referral from their primary care clinician prior to being seen. Another common issue that arises relates to the matching of the patient's insurance with that contracted by the provider. If the patient reveals that they are insured under ABC Health Plan, for example, but the clinician with whom they are scheduled is not a participating provider, the patient may be contacted to discuss financial arrangements. Depending on the size of the organization, these financial issues may be routed to a specific team of employees to address with the patient.

- **Orders.** Technology can be deployed to initiate actions based on the patient's reason for visit. If a patient is scheduled for a well-male physical examination, for example, an order set for labs is triggered in the EHR system. The patient can then proceed to the lab for the routine blood work associated with the physical examination and the results be communicated to the physician in advance of the patient's appointment.

- **Communication Platform.** Many ambulatory practices have a patient portal, which acts as a platform for secure communication between the practice and patients. Patients may grant portal access to their family members and caregivers so that they can easily obtain the patient's medical records. (There are legal considerations regarding access to health records, which should be reviewed and addressed by the practice prior to deploying a communication platform as compliance with current rules and regulations is of utmost importance.) The functions of a portal vary based on the technology, but the pre-arrival process is an opportune time to ensure that the patient is registered for the portal. This may be addressed during the appointment scheduling process, or an alert may be communicated after the appointment is reserved, but prior to the patient's arrival. The portal offers an opportunity for asynchronous communication, allowing for greater efficiency compared to traditional telecommunication means.

■   **Appointment Confirmation.** The practice may transmit communication to the patient via the portal, text, or call regarding the patient's upcoming appointment. This may serve as a confirmation of the time and date, but also may include instructions for the patient or other details about the appointment.

Increasingly, careful attention is paid to ensuring that clinical details related to the appointment and the patient's financial health are resolved prior to the patient's arrival.

Appointment Schedule

The backbone of an ambulatory practice is its appointment schedule. The appointment schedule serves three main purposes: access (efficient allocation of demand), workflow (efficient organization of supporting resources), and capacity management (efficient allocation of supply). A well-managed ambulatory setting is reliant upon a well-designed scheduling process to ensure resources are used efficiently, capacity is managed to best accommodate patient needs, and provider time is fully utilized in a productive manner.

Managing patient demand in the ambulatory practice setting is unique in that it is irregular and unpredictable. As an inpatient in a hospital or a resident in a nursing home, the patient is stationary. Demand can be fulfilled at the convenience of all parties without having to be concerned about the presence of the patient. In a hospital or a nursing home, the patient's presence is known. In the ambulatory setting, demand must be proactively anticipated and managed. Patient demand for ambulatory practice services is achieved by offering appointment slots to patients. Patients are given a certain time to arrive and be serviced. Therefore, the appointment schedule provides the opportunity for an effective allocation of demand that meets the capacity of the ambulatory practice.

The schedule not only defines time—patient availability based on day of the week and time of day combined with the corresponding appointment time slots—but it also provides the framework for servicing the patient. Therefore, the schedule informs who will deliver the care, the physical resources required for the services, and the support infrastructure. Once consisting of a spiral-bound notebook with a series of time slots accompanied by a jar of White-Out to facilitate any changes, the appointment schedule of today's ambulatory practice is automated. It is complex and sophisticated yet nimble and accommodating in order to address the efficient organization of supporting resources.

A clinician's time is the most valuable asset of an ambulatory practice; the time a clinician allocates to provide clinical care effectively defines "provider supply." The schedule provides a framework to efficiently allocate the supply of providers' time. If, for example, a patient fails to arrive for their appointment, the time allocated by the clinician to see the patient is lost, as there is no time to identify, contact, and arrange for another patient to be seen in real time. See the sidebar "Best Practice Scheduling Technique." Because the ambulatory practice relies on perishable inventory, capacity must be managed effectively. The best means of accomplishing the optimal delivery of provider supply is through the appointment schedule.

BEST PRACTICE SCHEDULING TECHNIQUE: STRATEGIC BOOKING

Strategic booking is the key to managing limited capacity in an efficient manner. Consider these three techniques to optimize the schedule of an ambulatory practice by strategic booking.

Predictive booking

Overbooking appointment slots throughout the day can translate into maintaining the desired daily patient volume. But if not done with care, overbooking can be disastrous to workflow. Instead, evaluate the characteristics of patients who fail to keep appointments (gender, insurance coverage, new versus established, etc.) and the nature of the appointment itself (day of week, time of day, procedure versus office visit, etc.). Overbook just those slots that predictably will not show. For example, you may find that new patients who were seen following unassigned weekend call at the hospital with post-discharge appointments on Monday mornings have a significantly higher no-show rate than any other category of patient. You could safely double-book those patients. Focus on predictable no-shows, such as a patient who has missed two previously scheduled appointments or double-book a "quick" visit to minimize the disruption if both patients arrive. If there is no pattern, overbook slots at the top of the hour—how many hours depends on the extent of the problem.

Level load

Next, recognize peaks of patient demand. Ambulatory practices experience ebbs and flows in patient volume; many practices find that Mondays are the busiest day of the week others tend to see seasonal shifts in demand. Whether it is a day, a week, a month, or a season, make sure that your schedule reflects this predictable fluctuation in demand. If you expect an influx of children to be seen for school physicals in August, make a temporary adjustment in your schedule to echo those expectations. Do not assume that the schedule is static; make adjustments to best match the providers' time with your patients' needs in order to successfully level load your schedule—and keep it running on time. Level load the schedule to aim for making resources available to match expected demand.

Horizon management

Finally, take strides to manage the scheduling horizon. The scheduling horizon—the lead time to an appointment—is a predictor of arrival rates. Research has demonstrated that every 30-day delay in the scheduling horizon increases the probability of nonarrivals by 11% (primary care) to 16% (specialty) (Woodcock et al., 2020). By analyzing and managing the scheduling horizon, a practice can improve the utilization of providers' time.

Use technology to assist in analyzing the opportunity—and perhaps even to implement a solution to it.

The framework for an appointment schedule in an ambulatory practice is often referred to as the scheduling **template**. Managing the scheduling template is considered crucial to effectively meet the goal of getting the right patient to the right provider at the right time. Therefore, it is common for an ambulatory practice to employ personnel dedicated to managing the schedule. In large ambulatory practices, full-time staff members often have the title of "scheduling architect," "master scheduler," "template builder," or "capacity manager." A 1:100 ratio of schedule management personnel compared to clinicians is common.

There are typically two elements to an appointment schedule—a "master" template and a "daily" or "session" template. For example, a gastroenterologist holds clinic every Tuesday and Thursday from 8:00 a.m. to 5:00 p.m. with a 60-minute lunch break. Her template contains eight 30-minute new patient slots, and sixteen 15-minute established patient slots. This is her master template. Next week, her daughter has a school play at 4:00 p.m. on Thursday. Therefore, the slots from 4:00 to 5:00 p.m. are blocked to ensure that she can have the time off—and her patients are not inconvenienced by arriving at 4:00 p.m. without a physician to see them. While her master template remains, a change is made to the schedule on next Thursday. Another scenario is that there may be a patient with special needs presenting to the gastroenterology clinic next Thursday. This requires the physician to examine the patient, consult with the patient's caregivers, and confer with other providers about the patient. In this scenario, despite the patient being an established patient, a 30-minute appointment window is needed instead of the usual 15-minute period. This would not be consistent with the master template, thereby requiring the next 15-minute slot to be blocked to have the appropriate time for the patient. These examples illustrate the necessity of having a consistent "master" schedule while also having the flexibility to address the allocation of time to accommodate the providers' daily schedule.

An ambulatory practice must actively manage the template by regularly reviewing for changes and adjusting as needed, minimally once per year, or at least quarterly. An ambulatory practice may manage the build and maintenance of all aspects of the appointment template centrally—or there may be a main effort to manage the masters, but local personnel (e.g., the physician) may manage the nuances of the day.

To effectively manage the daily, temporary changes, the schedule may allow for blocks, holds, and freezes. The terminology may be specific to the practice's technology vendor; however, the functionalities of blocking a portion of the schedule, holding a slot for a designated purpose, or freezing a slot as nonschedulable are often provided by the system for temporary edits to the schedule. Because they remove slots from the pool of schedulable time, an ambulatory practice may introduce rules related to the blocks, holds, and freezes. For example, a multispecialty practice may choose to hold slots on the dermatologists' schedule to accommodate rapid access to internal referrals for patients sent for consultations by the practice's internists. If the slot being held is not used within two business days of the appointment, however, it is released back into the pool to schedule any patient appointment. Ambulatory practices with effective schedule management may accompany a "release" strategy in the event of blocks, holds, and freezes, particularly ones that are permanent.

On the schedule, appointment slots may be in the form of type or time. For example, if appointment type is used, there may be slots allocated to "physical," "new patient," "established patient," and "same-day urgent" visits. Some practices have established hundreds of appointment types from which to choose; others have moved to a simple model with a limited number of types—for example, "short" and "long"—with the explanation documented in the EHR system regarding the reason for visit.

The duration of appointments may be 15 minutes (to signal an appointment of short time duration, often reserved for established patients) and 30 minutes (for long appointments, for new patients). The appointments are often reported as durations of time and may vary by specialty. For example, a multispecialty ambulatory practice may have a 15/30 template for its neurologists, which would signal appointment slots are 15 and 30 minutes; a 10/20 for its pediatricians; a 20/40 for its endocrinologists, and so forth. Table 5.1 presents benchmarks for **appointment durations** by specialty.

In determining the appointment durations, it is crucial to ensure that time is not wasted. Figure 5.2 demonstrates two templates for the first hour of the day, 8:00 a.m. to 9:00 a.m.—the first one is not well managed with only 45 of 60 available minutes booked; the other is well managed with 60 of 60 minutes booked using a standard 10/20 duration model.

Another template strategy is to offer consistent time slots throughout the day, such as every 15 minutes or every 20 minutes, with the notion that some patient visits will be of short duration and others of longer duration; however, the preciseness of this designation often cannot be forecasted based on the patient's chief complaint. Instead, the clinicians and support staff work flexibly to accommodate patients throughout the clinic session.

For some specialties, there is little clinical information needed from patients to book an appointment beyond their chief complaint. For others, extensive details must be extracted to create a visit itinerary. As an example, for oncology patients, this may include a test, an infusion, therapy, or other service before or after the encounter with the clinician. Most appointments fall in the middle, requiring the patient to provide sufficient detail for the scheduler to locate the right clinician at the right time while not overwhelming either the scheduler or the patient.

An appointment schedule in an ambulatory practice is much like playing a game of Tetris®, the tile-matching video game created in the 1980s. Most practices utilize technology to aid in the scheduling process; templates are created and maintained electronically. Template management is supplemented by readily available technological solutions such as provider matching, automated **self-scheduling**, and **wait lists**, described herein.

TABLE 5.1 Median Appointment Duration Benchmarks by Specialty (in minutes)

SPECIALTY	ESTABLISHED PATIENTS	NEW PATIENTS
ALLERGY/IMMUNOLOGY	20.0	40.0
DERMATOLOGY	15.0	20.0
CARDIOLOGY	25.0	40.0
ENDOCRINOLOGY	20.0	40.0
INFECTIOUS DISEASE	20.0	40.0
INTERNAL MEDICINE	30.0	40.0
GASTROENTEROLOGY	30.0	30.0
HEMATOLOGY	20.0	60.0
MEDICAL ONCOLOGY	30.0	60.0
NEPHROLOGY	20.0	40.0
NEUROLOGY	30.0	60.0
OBSTETRICS/GYNECOLOGY	15.0	30.0
OPHTHALMOLOGY	15.0	15.5
ORAL AND MAXILLOFACIAL SURGERY	30.0	30.0
OTOLARYNGOLOGY	15.0	30.0
PAIN	20.0	40.0
PHYSIATRY	20.0	40.0
PODIATRY	15.0	30.0
PSYCHIATRY	30.0	60.0
PULMONARY MEDICINE	30.0	45.0
RHEUMATOLOGY	20.0	40.0
SURGERY: CARDIOVASCULAR	20.0	30.0
SURGERY: COLORECTAL	15.0	30.0
SURGERY: GENERAL	15.0	30.0
SURGERY: NEURO	20.5	30.0
SURGERY: ORTHOPEDICS	15.0	30.0
SURGERY: PLASTICS	15.0	30.0
SURGERY: VASCULAR	15.0	30.0
SURGICAL ONCOLOGY	20.0	30.0
UROLOGY	15.0	30.0

SOURCE: Patient Access Collaborative 2021 based on 2020 data. Median data.

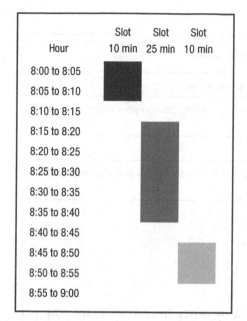 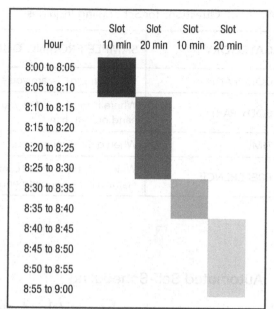

FIGURE 5.2 Appointment template examples.

Provider Matching

In a large, multispecialty practice, it is difficult to deploy an effective strategy to manually manage the three elements of the schedule: access, workflow, and capacity. Scheduling is often centralized to capture economies of scale, improve service, and better distribute supply across an ambulatory enterprise. The consequence is a challenge related to scheduling, as aptly described by the practicing physician and informaticist, Dr. Jonathan Teich, in an interview with the *American Medical News* in 2004: "Mabel is the generic scheduling administrator who has been working for Dr. Smith for 35 years, and knows a thousand nuances and idiosyncrasies and preferences that have been silently established over the years. . . . Unfortunately for the computer world, it's extremely difficult to find out what Mabel really knows, let alone try and put it into an algorithm" (Versel, 2004). Technology in the form of integrated provider matching solutions, automated scheduling decision trees, and customer relationship management solutions have risen to address the "Mabel factor." For example, the ambulatory practice can create a decision tree featuring questions that guide a patient to the correct provider on the basis of the patient's responses. The algorithm may include probing questions that offer information about a multitude of factors (see Table 5.2).

The solutions focus on allowing ambulatory practices to leverage centralized management without sacrificing the value of marrying the patients' or referring clinicians' stated needs with the correct provider, time, and location.

TABLE 5.2 Questions for Scheduling Inquiries

CATEGORY	SAMPLE PROBING QUESTIONS
COMPLAINT	What symptom(s) are you experiencing?
BODY PART	Where is the pain? Are you experiencing pain in your right hand or left hand or both hand?
TIME	When did the injury occur?
PREFERENCE	Which location is most convenient for you, or are you looking for the first available appointment?

Automated Self-Scheduling

Reservation systems have been widely adopted by other industries managing perishable inventory, to include airlines, hotels, and restaurants. With solutions that allow improvements in the management of the schedule, ambulatory practices are adopting tools to place the responsibility for scheduling in patients' hands. Self-scheduling offers benefits to the practice by reducing labor costs. The opportunity to self-schedule may be deployed via the practice's portal, offered as a solution disseminated to patients solely for the purpose of self-scheduling, or provided through a relationship with a third-party scheduling service. For patients, the convenience of scheduling an appointment 24 hours a day, seven days a week is significant. Some ambulatory practices choose to allow any patient to schedule; others restrict self-scheduling to patients seeking appointments for certain services (e.g., screening mammograms), to patients who are established with the practice, and to patients needing particular appointment types (e.g., follow-up appointments). Patients may choose to self-schedule, or the practice may proactively push a notification to the patient with instructions to schedule an appointment (e.g., "It's time to schedule your flu shot!").

Wait Lists

Scheduling churn occurs as an appointment date draws close: Patients may cancel or reschedule, or providers may alter their time commitment. This runway of time provides opportunity for the ambulatory practice to rebook newly opened slots. The appointments may be brokered via schedulers handling patients who call for an appointment or through the self-scheduling platform. Practices may also benefit from wait lists. These lists may be maintained manually, documenting patients who desire appointments at an earlier time. A more efficient method is an automated wait list. When an appointment becomes available due to a change generated by the patient or provider, an alert about the open slot is communicated automatically to a preestablished number of patients for a predetermined amount of time. For example, an open slot tomorrow in the orthopedic practice would trigger a text to 10 patients, allowing them one hour before another 10 patients are alerted to the open slot. The communication would direct patients to select the open slot, with the first to respond capturing it. The practice may reduce or expand the number of patients who receive the communication, as well as the timing, depending on the response rate. Another effective method to improve the utilization rate of the appointment slots is to proactively push communications to patients due for a service. For example, an internal medicine practice with a newly opened slot may reach out to a patient due for their "Welcome to Medicare" exam.

The technological solutions related to scheduling offer a means of enhancing the scheduling process. Increasingly, practices are using novel product offerings to supplement their workflows related to provider matching, automated self-scheduling, and wait list management.

Appointment Confirmations

The ideal state for an ambulatory practice is to have all patients arrive for their booked appointments. Although nonarrivals cannot be fully prevented, appointment confirmations may improve the probability of arrival. Depending on the lag time between the scheduling transaction—that is, when the patient scheduled the appointment—and the appointment date, a confirmation may be communicated hours, days, or weeks in advance of the appointment. The communication may occur via text, phone, secure electronic message or a combination of methods. The ambulatory practice may decide to confirm the appointment, as well as communicate instructions, directions, fees, or other important details about the appointment.

Time is the greatest asset of an ambulatory practice, with the appointment schedule serving as its backbone for allocating patient demand for care efficiently. Therefore, key performance indicators (KPIs) have been established to quantitatively measure a facility's effectiveness in schedule management. The ability to measure a facility's performance with the scheduling process promotes accountability as well as informs actionable steps to improve the scheduling process. Metrics to monitor scheduling vary by ambulatory practice based on factors such as the specialty, size, and ability to capture and report the data. KPIs are shown in Table 5.3.

Referrals

The term *referral* in an ambulatory practice has two distinct meanings: an insurance referral and a referral for clinical care.

An insurance referral is a mechanism deployed by an insurance company to manage demand for services that consists of a formal request for a patient to be seen.

TABLE 5.3 Key Performance Indicators in Ambulatory Scheduling Management

NEW PATIENT LAG TIME - SCHEDULED PATIENTS	The median span of time, as measured in calendar days, between the date of a new patient's appointment request (e.g., telephone call, portal-based request, referring physician on behalf of the patient, etc.) and the date of the appointment, for all providers with an active template in your scheduling system. Report this based on a retrospective view of a minimum period of 90 days during the reporting period. Note that this is the median number of calendar days between the request and the appointment schedule. The status of the patient's arrival is not relevant to this metric.
NEW PATIENT LAG TIME - ARRIVED PATIENTS	The median span of time, as measured in calendar days, between the date of a new patient's appointment request (e.g., telephone call, portal-based request, referring physician on behalf of the patient, etc.) and the date of the encounter, for all providers with an active template in your scheduling system. Report this based on a retrospective view of a minimum period of 90 days during the reporting period. Note that this is the median number of calendar days between the request and the encounter. The status of the patient's arrival is vital to this metric; only report those patients who arrived.
PERCENTAGE OF NEW PATIENTS SCHEDULED WITHIN 14 DAYS	The percentage of new patients scheduled within 14 calendar days of their appointment request, during the reporting period. Include all patients who were scheduled regardless of whether they rescheduled, cancelled or did not showed.
PERCENTAGE OF NEW PATIENTS ARRIVED WITHIN 14 DAYS	The percentage of new patients arrived (i.e., seen) within 14 calendar days of their appointment request, during the reporting period. Include only patients who arrived.
FILL RATE	The percentage of providers' time in clinic that is filled with arrived patients, as defined by the arrived time in clinic (sum of appointment duration for arrivals), expressed as a percentage of the total allocated time on providers' daily schedules (sum of appointment duration available for booking) during the reporting period. Report on *all* patients (i.e., not only "new" patients). Time may be measured in minutes, hours, or appointment slots.
PERCENTAGE SCHEDULED, BUT NOT ARRIVED	Total = The Sum of No-Show, Cancel, Bump, and Other, based on the total percentage of patients who are given a scheduled appointment (includes same-day appointments that are scheduled) but do not arrive. The denominator includes *all* scheduled appointments (i.e., not only "new" patients). The reasons for non-arrival may include no-shows, advance/last-minute cancelations, provider-initiated bumps or other reasons. Note that these slots may have been refilled, but the rate is to recognize rework in addition to capacity opportunities. Report this based on a retrospective view of a minimum period of 90 days during the reporting period, with the end of the period at least 30 days from today's date (in order to ensure that missing charges/open charts are accounted for). No-show: Patient fails to present for their scheduled appointment without any advance notification, as defined by the institution. Cancel: Patient provides advance notification that they canceled a scheduled appointment, as defined by the institution. Bump: Physician/provider cancels a patient's scheduled appointment, as defined by the institution. Other: Pending (e.g., chart not closed), other. Report percentages of total volume, not actual volume. The total of the percentages should equal your nonarrival rate.

(continued)

TABLE 5.3 Key Performance Indicators in Ambulatory Scheduling Management
(*Continued*)

REFERRAL CONVERSION RATE	The proportion, as expressed as a percentage, of inbound internal and external referrals that are converted to scheduled appointments. Denominator equals all received appointment requests from a referring provider, regardless of transmission method (i.e., referrals for care that may be received by internal order, external fax, Health Information Exchange); the numerator equals all of said referrals that result in an appointment being scheduled. Include all referrals regardless of insurance status (e.g., if the referral was for a noncovered service that may or may not be "authorized" by insurance, it should be included as it is a referral for care), and all appointments regardless of arrival status (i.e., if the patient does not show, the patient is still counted as the appointment was scheduled). Report on all patients (i.e., not only "new" patients). Include all outpatient services for which data are tracked, with the exception of laboratory and imaging (e.g., ambulatory physician/provider encounters only). Do not include laboratory or imaging orders.
REFERRAL TURNAROUND TIME - PATIENT CONTACT	The proportion, as expressed as a percentage, of referrals in which the patient is contacted within two calendar days of the referral being logged into the referral management system. Referral Request Definition: any documented request for an appointment from a referring provider that is logged into the EHR, practice management system that is converted to an actionable status through the creation of a referral record. Inclusion/Exclusion Criteria: *Include* all referral requests regardless of transmission method (i.e. order, phone, fax, direct message, web platform, etc.). *Exclude* self-referral phone calls where the creation of the appointment request and the patient contact are occurring at the same time (e.g., some health systems create referral records for inbound phone requests from the patient-facing vanity line. In that situation, the referral request and patient contact are one in the same). Notes: For ease and practicality of reporting, the time frame being reported is from the time the referral is logged into the referral management system until the first documented contact attempt to the patient. By this definition, any time prior to referral being entered into the referral management system is excluded (e.g., if a referral sits on a fax server for 24 hours prior to being entered into the referral management system, then that time is excluded). A contact attempt is any documented attempt to reach the patient (phone call, text message, message through patient portal, etc.). This metric pertains to the contact, not the appointment date (i.e., this should not represent the percentage of patients scheduled and/or seen within two calendar days).
REFERRAL TURNAROUND TIME - SCHEDULING TRANSACTION	The proportion, as expressed as a percentage, of referrals in which the patient has been granted a scheduled appointment within two calendar days of the referral being logged into the referral management system. Referral Request Definition: any documented request for an appointment from a referring provider that is logged into the EHR, practice management system that is converted to an actionable status through the creation of a referral record.

(*continued*)

TABLE 5.3 Key Performance Indicators in Ambulatory Scheduling Management (*Continued*)

	Inclusion/exclusion criteria: *Include* all referral requests regardless of transmission method (i.e. order, phone, fax, direct message, web platform, etc.). *Exclude* self-referral phone calls where the creation of the appointment request and the patient contact are occurring at the same time (e.g., some health systems create referral records for inbound phone requests from the patient-facing vanity line. In that situation, the referral request and patient contact are one in the same).
	Notes: For ease and practicality of reporting, the time frame being reported is from the time the referral is logged into the referral management system until the first documented contact attempt to the patient. By this definition, any time prior to referral being entered into the referral management system is excluded (for example, if a referral sits on a fax server for 24 hours prior to being entered into the referral management system, then that time is excluded). This metric pertains to the appointment being granted, not the appointment date (i.e., this should not represent the scheduling transaction, not the percentage of patients seen within two calendar days).

SOURCE: Patient Access Collaborative 2021 (used with permission).

A referral may be issued by the patient's primary care provider or specialist depending on the nature of the referral. Depending on the insurance company and referral type, it may or may not require insurance company review.

The insurance company sets the parameters for the referral, including the process and timing. It is common for primary care clinicians to receive referrals electronically and require 24 to 48 hours to process. If care is provided by the specialist without a required referral, insurance payment for the clinical services is not assured. Some insurers may issue guidelines to primary care physicians about issuing referrals, with a minority tying financial risk to the process. In this manner, the insurance company is leveraging the referral process via the primary care clinician to control service and resource utilization (see the sidebar "Insurance Referrals" for additional information about insurance referrals).

The second type of referral is a referral for clinical care, typically from primary care clinician to a specialist. If it is accompanied by the term *transfer*, the primary care clinician is granting another party the responsibility for the patient's care and is typically no longer involved or involved only peripherally. Some specialty practices require *all* patients to have a referral to receive an appointment. Patients are told: "A Referral is Required." Other than the insurance policies that necessitate insurance referrals, this is a self-imposed request. Much like the insurance company, the specialty practice is controlling utilization by requesting that all patients be referred by a primary care clinician. This may be a function of desiring patients to be managed by the primary care clinician, wanting patients to be evaluated and triaged for appropriateness of specialty care, and/or having demand that exceeds the specialty practice's capacity (thereby building in a time lag), which may result in rationing care.

INSURANCE REFERRALS

Insurance companies may impose requirements regarding the approval for care. In an ambulatory practice, it is common for referrals and **prior authorizations** to be mandatory. These advance approvals are reviewed for medical necessity.

Referral. This is a process through which the primary care physician permits or instructs a patient to obtain a service or item from another physician or other provider. A referral provides approval by the patient's primary care physician for them to access a specialist. The referral may incorporate the number of visits, time frame, and type of services.

Prior Authorization. Through this process, the physician obtains advance approval from the patient's insurance company to receive a service or item; also known as pre-service authorization request. A review of medical necessity may be required for certain procedures, drugs, items, and/or supplies. The ordering physician is typically responsible for obtaining the prior authorization; the entity rendering the service is accountable for confirming the authorization has been obtained. The patient is not responsible for acquiring the authorization. A referral may also be required to accompany the authorization.

Medical necessity is determined by the insurance company, not the provider, for the purposes of insurance coverage. Each company maintains its own definition, which are typically found in the insurer's provider manual. The Centers for Medicare and Medicaid Services (2020b), which administers the Medicare program, defines an item or service to be "reasonable and necessary" if it meets the criteria listed herein:

1. It is safe and effective;
2. It is not experimental or investigational; and
3. It is appropriate, including the duration and frequency in terms of whether the service or item is:
   - Furnished in accordance with accepted standards of medical practice for the diagnosis or treatment of the beneficiary's condition or to improve the function of a malformed body member;
   - Furnished in a setting appropriate to the beneficiary's medical needs and condition;
   - Ordered and furnished by qualified personnel; and,
   - One that meets, but does not exceed, the beneficiary's medical need. (Section 3.6.2.2)

Guidelines for referrals and prior authorizations differ by payer, by plan, and over time. Ambulatory practices must maintain currency regarding requirements to ensure accurate and timely payment. Complying with the requirements also facilitates the patient's financial health; referrals and authorizations ensure claims are adjudicated correctly, thereby avoiding inaccurate patient financial responsibility.

Regardless of the type of referral (insurance or clinical care), dedicated personnel are typically assigned to fulfill these requests. These personnel accept and process requests by patients and by specialty practices communicating on their behalf. The often-called "referral coordinators" ensure the necessary data are collected regarding the referral and coordinate with the insurance company and patient to secure required authorizations.

To avoid a referral process creating a barrier to care, it is essential to understand why and when referrals are required by the practice. If referrals are required for all patients, it is crucial to communicate with patients and referral sources about the mechanics of the process. Some practices have used electronic consults ("eConsults") successfully, automating the communication between the primary care clinician and the specialist. This may be accompanied by an algorithm-driven order related to the referral, wherein the primary care clinician is inputting specific data about the patient such as a test result. Some ambulatory practices that include primary care and specialists perform these consults on a real-time basis; should the consult indicate that a referral is in order, it is facilitated at that time. Short of an electronic process, some practices have designed formal work processes between primary care and specialists. These agreed-on processes (often referred to as "compacts") outline the referral process in detail so that all parties understand how to facilitate a referral.

Stage 2: Arrival

The second stage of ambulatory practice operations is the patient arrival to the practice for their scheduled encounter. Patients may present exactly at the specified date and time, but it is more common for patients to arrive early. Researchers at Johns Hopkins University found that of 1,500 patients, 90.7% arrived early, averaging 24.1 minutes in advance of their appointments (Williams et al., 2014). Scheduling in the ambulatory setting involves people, so care must be given to managing patients that may come before, at, or after their preset appointment times. With dozens, perhaps hundreds of patients arriving in a single day for their appointment, it is critical to have a process to streamline the patient arrival process.

The patient arrival stage is composed of three steps: check-in, rooming, and **clinical intake**, each of which are described in the following subsections.

Check In

The patient arriving for their appointment in the ambulatory setting may be met by a designated person(s) who "checks in" the patient. This process may be fully performed by the staff member who greets the patient, often referred to as the receptionist or patient services representative, or it may involve employing technological tools; as examples, a tablet may be handed to a patient or the patient may be directed to a self-check-in kiosk. Regardless of how it is performed, patients are typically asked to confirm the registration details provided at the scheduling process, such as name, address, date of birth, and insurance information. Consistent with the phone-based interaction that occurs with the patient, patients are typically identified by a minimum of two data elements. The patient may also be asked to provide payment for the visit, for example, the patient's out-of-pocket costs, such as their copayment.

Furthermore, this process may involve the collection of medical information to include additional details about the patient's concern(s), medical history, and past social and family history. Furthermore, patients may be asked to sign forms to acknowledge compliance with the practice's policies, as well as requirements from insurance companies, and state and federal regulations. Exhibit 5.1 lists forms commonly collected during the arrival process, noting that the list of common forms should not be construed as a comprehensive guide. Well-managed practices recognize and comply with current requirements related to notifications, acknowledgments, and requirements in accordance with state and federal law.

Some elements of the arrival process have shifted to the pre-encounter. Increasingly, practices have enabled technology solutions to allow information to be collected in advance, allowing patients to self–"check in" before their appointment. If this information is gathered prior to the appointment, the arrival process may be limited to a brief confirmation of the patient's arrival, perhaps by the patient's physical presence in the reception area, a text from their phone, or confirmation of arrival on a kiosk.

Once the patient completes the designated check in process, there is typically an internal mechanism to alert the clinical personnel in the practice that a patient arrived for the scheduled appointment. This is most commonly integrated in the practice's EHR system but may also involve a visual cue that is signaled, such as an exam room flag or light. The process itself may consist of multiple alerts, such as the clinical personnel first informed that the patient has arrived for their appointment, with a second alert that signals that the patient has completed the arrival process and is ready to be roomed. The arrival process differs by ambulatory practice, however, internal compliance to a consistent process is crucial. Otherwise, the patient may remain in the reception area or exam room for prolonged periods as no one has been alerted that the patient is ready to be seen or ready for the next step in the visit process.

Rooming

After the patient arrives for their scheduled appointment and an alert has been given to the clinical personnel that the check-in process is complete, an employee prepares the exam room and materials required for the encounter with the patient. Once this is complete, the employee—typically a medical assistant—meets the patient in the reception area, escorts the patient to the exam room, conducts clinical intake, and prepares the patient for the provider portion of the encounter. There may be

EXHIBIT 5.1 COMMON FORMS USED DURING PATIENT ARRIVAL

Assignment of benefits form: The patient (or guarantor on the account) agrees to assign insurance benefits to the practice so the practice may bill and receive payment on the patient's behalf. The form is typically signed for all new patients, upon changes in insurance for existing patients, and each annum.

Medical records release form: The patient agrees to permit the practice to release medical records on their behalf to third parties. This includes medical documentation requested by insurance companies when a claim is disputed.

Waiver form: The patient is informed of the expectation regarding the financial responsibility for services for which the insurance company will not cover. The Centers for Medicare and Medicaid Services maintains a form specific to Medicare beneficiaries: Advance Beneficiary Notice (ABN). An ABN is a written notification made to a Medicare beneficiary at the point of care before items or services are furnished for which the physician believes that Medicare will decline to cover.

Financial and administrative policies form: The patient is informed of the practice's policies regarding billing and collections, appointments, prescription renewals and refills, communications, and referrals. These may include details about the protocols for such processes (e.g., when statements are transmitted), penalties for noncompliance (e.g., no-show fee), and time frames (e.g., prescription renewals take 24 hours).

Notice of Privacy Practices: The privacy regulations of the Health Insurance Portability and Accountability Act of 1996 require physicians who have a direct treatment relationship with an individual to document and convey a notice of privacy practices. The patient is requested to acknowledge receipt of the notice.

Patient history form: Data are gathered from the patient regarding the patient's medical, social, and family history. The information collected may be consistent across all physicians and specialties (e.g., history of smoking); it may be supplemented by questions specific to the specialty or chief complaint of the patient.

a designated employee to retrieve the patient—or there may be a pool of personnel facilitating patient retrieval and rooming, working fluidly throughout the day to ensure the patients are retrieved, roomed, and readied for the provider encounter.

Personnel duties may also involve checking to ensure the room and/or equipment is sanitized, locating a tablet or computer to record information, or walking to the reception area to retrieve the patient. Although it is commonplace to state the patient's name loudly upon reaching the reception area; as an alternative, practices can retrieve the patient's picture as a component of their record so the employee may personally approach the patient in the reception area and escort the patient to an exam room. In an ambulatory practice, escorting the patient to the exam room area is often referred to as bringing the patient "to the back."

Although the patient may obediently follow the medical assistant or other clinical associate, this is an opportunity to engage with the patient in a meaningful, service-oriented manner. To accomplish this, the employee should introduce themselves, confirm the patient's identity to assure the correct patient is being escorted to the back, and ask the patient if they require any assistance in moving to the exam area. Staff must be cognizant of any patient limitations and should not make assumptions about a patient's abilities. For example, it is best practice to walk alongside patients when escorting them rather than in front of them to keep the patient in view.

Escorting the patient can be a valuable opportunity to observe patient behavior and learn more about their needs. The patient may be in pain, scared, or experiencing emotions that may leave him or her in a vulnerable and unsteady state. Engaging with the patient offers an opportunity to express empathy and demonstrate compassion and concern for the patient experience. This focus on the patient experience is critical in the well-managed ambulatory setting.

Clinical Intake

Each ambulatory practice should develop a formal clinical intake process that is consistent across like specialties and yet sufficiently flexible to address patient-specific needs, such as the collection of vital signs and other clinical preparation needed for the encounter with the provider. For example, a patient's weight may be captured for a patient who is scheduled to see an internist, while that step may be skipped for a patient destined for the ophthalmologist. For some multispecialty practices, the process consists of an intake checklist that is the same for every clinician. Clinical intake may involve capturing and documenting vitals such as height, weight, and blood pressure; it may also entail asking questions of the patient or administering a health screening.

A consistent clinical intake process assures optimal compliance, which reduces confusion and enhances quality and safety within the practice. The level of effectiveness of the clinical intake portion of the encounter within an ambulatory setting can also have a positive or negative impact to the practice's quality and performance, ultimately influencing value-based payments and related incentive programs. For example, during the clinical intake process, key questions related to various quality indicators (e.g., influenza vaccination) may be asked and the results documented. The consistency of the clinical intake process assures all patients proceed through the same process and all data are captured. A thoughtfully designed clinical intake process can also enhance efficiency, minimizing wasted time and unnecessary resource utilization.

Clinical intake may include what is commonly referred to as "**standing orders**." Typically triggered by the patient's diagnosis or presenting concern, the order may include collecting a specimen for a test or proceeding with the performance of the test. For example, if a patient has a visibly deformed arm following an accident, the patient may be taken for an x-ray of the arm during the clinical intake process. There may be standing orders that are always applicable—for example, requesting that pregnant patients provide a urine sample. The patient's time is preserved by proceeding with a specimen collection or test that will be rendered. In doing so, the results can be known more expeditiously to guide the care and treatment plan espoused by the clinician.

Consider the clinical intake process as that which prepares the patient for the next step, which is archetypally the face-to-face (F2F) visit between the patient and the clinician. Once completed, the designated personnel member alerts the provider that the patient is ready. The signaling is often performed electronically, through the EHR system. The alert may be supplemented with a visual indication of the step—a flag, a magnet, or a sign on the door, which may offer a quick and efficient cue of the next patient to be seen. Additional cues may be established for other activities, to include, as examples, that an order is waiting or a result is ready.

Depending on the size of the ambulatory practice, there may be one—or many— personnel participating in clinical intake. The process is either staffed by allocating personnel to work with a specific clinician or assigned as a team to support several clinicians. Alternatively, there may be a pool of personnel who perform the intake on a rotational basis. Regardless of the method of staffing, well-managed practices consider the importance of reducing patients' wait time and streamlining the flow of patients for the clinician. Consider this process like airplanes taking off and landing; indeed, some large practices invest in the position of a patient flow coordinator to act like an air traffic controller.

Stage 3: Encounter

After receiving the alert that the patient is ready to be seen, the physician, advanced practice provider, or other healthcare professional readies for the encounter. In a well-managed ambulatory practice, the clinician will have reviewed the patient's chart prior to entering the exam room, either the day prior in preparation for the following day, at a morning "**huddle**" (or at both morning and midday huddles) with the clinical team in which key information is reviewed and visit preparation needs are communicated, or in the minutes before walking into the exam room (see the sidebar "Huddles" for additional information about huddles).

Increasingly, ambulatory practices are leveraging technology to aid in preparing for the patient's clinical encounter. For example, there may be a daily report of test results that have been received for patients who are scheduled to be seen, as well as results that remain outstanding, thus prompting someone to locate them. Furthermore, a report may be generated for patients on the schedule who have preventive

HUDDLES

Huddles are stand-up meetings performed once a day with a team, typically no more than 10 minutes. The goal for a huddle is to be an effective and efficient tool for communicating about incoming patients and the flow of the clinic session (UCSF Center for Excellence in Primary Care, 2013). Huddles allow the well-managed ambulatory practice to prepare for personnel changes and anticipate the needs of patients, thereby avoiding surprises to permit the practice to operate efficiently and effectively (Yu, 2015). The huddle may include all personnel in the practice, a subset of the practice, or a teamlet (e.g., the clinical and medical assistant). The composition of the huddle depends on the size of the practice; when determining the construct of huddles, well-managed ambulatory practices recognize that engaging everyone in problem identification and resolution is critical. Huddles enable participants to look back to assess performance and to look forward to proactively flag concerns (Institute for Healthcare Improvement [IHI], n.d.).

services that are due. The huddle is an opportune time to review these reports and to consider other aspects of preparedness: Is the equipment ready for Mr. Smith? Is the interpreter scheduled for Ms. Sanjay? Are there appropriate accommodations for Mr. Martìnez, who has a mobility issue? Running through the patients on the schedule during the huddle provides an invaluable opportunity to prepare, thereby promoting efficiency.

Alternatively, an ambulatory practice may not have a daily huddle. In these instances, there may be no time set aside in advance for individual or team preparation; the clinician may walk into the room and start asking the patient questions. This may result in needing assistance—to locate a test result, find an interpreter, and so forth. If the circumstances dictate, the clinician may perform the task required or seek the assistance of a medical assistant or other support personnel.

Encounters may last minutes—or hours. The steps of the encounter vary by specialty, clinician and patient; however, a helpful framework is that of SOAP, which stands for subjective, objective, assessment, and plan. Years ago, an encounter was documented in the form of a written SOAP note. Although such a note no longer exists in the electronic age, having been replaced by electronic templates, the framework is still valid for clinician/patient encounters in the ambulatory setting. Indeed, the visit templates for encounter documentation in the EHR system may still be organized in the SOAP format.

The encounter may be a consultation, examination, or procedure. The specifics of the patient's medical needs dictate the type of encounter, although typically ambulatory practices consider and prepare for common encounters. For example, a family medicine practice may have a standard provision for patients who present for a well-woman exam that includes a pelvic exam. The materials—lubricant, speculum, and so on—may be set up in the exam room prior to the patient's arrival in the room, in accordance with specifications established by the physicians, advanced practice providers and other members of the clinical team. Like many aspects of the ambulatory setting, the details vary, but a standard approach to the process that is applied in a consistent fashion is critical to an efficient, well-managed ambulatory practice.

Documentation of the Clinical Encounter

Timely and accurate documentation of the clinical encounter is required. The documentation provides a clear record of the patient's encounter, including treatments, outcomes, and future plans for care as appropriate. Accurate documentation also serves as the basis for coding and billing of clinical services.

Ideally, documentation of the clinical encounter is completed by the conclusion of the encounter. Clinicians may take notes during the encounter, leaving the final assessment and plan until the end of the visit. Others perform the documentation after the patient departs; post-encounter documentation may occur between every patient, following a group of patients, or at the conclusion of the clinic session. Still others hire personnel called "scribes" to take notes on their behalf during the encounter (and perhaps perform additional duties, such as retrieving equipment or assisting with a procedure). When a scribe documents the encounter, the clinician may review and sign off at the conclusion of the visit or later in the day. Considerations regarding the process and timing of documentation are critical.

A well-managed ambulatory practice features documentation that is accurate, timely and complete. According to the National Committee for Quality Assurance (NCQA, 2018), "consistent, current and complete documentation in the medical record is an essential component of quality patient care." The documentation provides a clear record of the encounter, which not only reflects the diagnosis, plan of care, and outcomes but also serves as a useful tool for reflecting recommendations, risks, decision-making, and patient expectations. The documentation also informs practice administrative and clinical personnel—internal or external—who may be working with the patient. If legal or other regulatory questions arise, documentation is the first step evaluated in identifying the care and treatment rendered to the patient.

The operations of an ambulatory practice may accommodate the documentation process by providing an office, workstation, or compact touch-down booth for the clinician to work. There may be time allotted in the schedule for documentation, or more often than not, time is embedded within the encounter but is not distinctly set aside on the schedule. As an example, a 20-minute appointment may involve 15 minutes of F2F visit time, with five minutes used for documentation and planning for next steps in the care and treatment plan for the patient.

Stage 4: Post-Encounter

The fourth stage of ambulatory practice operations—the post-encounter—may involve additional work prior to the patient leaving the practice. This can include processing an order for a laboratory, imaging study, or therapy; providing patient education; scheduling a procedure or surgery; and appointing the patient for a follow up visit. The post-encounter action also may incorporate a referral to another physician, advanced practice provider, or other healthcare professional in or outside of the ambulatory practice. In extenuating circumstances, an ambulance may be called to transport the patient to a hospital.

Depending on the action, the clinician may communicate with an employee to assist in the next step of the patient's care—or patients may be given instructions for subsequent activities to pursue on their own as part of a self-care protocol. For patients who are serviced in the practice, the issue of *where* to perform the action is an important consideration. If there are a multitude of exam rooms—more than are needed at any one time in the practice—then the patient may always be serviced in the exam room. Instead of being escorted or directed to a lab, for example, a phlebotomist may be called to the room, bringing the necessary equipment with them. Maintaining equipment on roving carts—the EKG machine, for example—streamlines this step.

If exam rooms are at a premium, which is often the case, the patient may be moved to a different area of the facility to complete the task or tasks. The circumstances will dictate the situation. If the patient needs a CT scan, for example, the patient would necessarily be escorted to the location of the machine. Even if equipment is not needed, the location of the action may be dictated by the patient's circumstances. If a patient has mobility issues, the practice may want to minimize travel to and from various areas in the practice, electing to keep the patient in the exam room and bring the services to the patient. If a patient was given a concerning diagnosis, for example, and a procedure needs to be scheduled, it may not be in the best interest of the patient's emotional well-being to move them back to the reception area to wait for a scheduler to be available. The scheduler should come to the exam room.

In general, tasks that can be performed rapidly such as scheduling follow-up visits are moved to a central processing area. Actions that involve mobile equipment, labor-intensive tasks, and the communication of sensitive information are performed by leaving the patient in the exam room and servicing them there—or escorting the patient to a designated area that offers space and privacy.

Like other elements in ambulatory practice operations, there is no single approach to the post-encounter. Availability, capacity, facility design, and placement of equipment and personnel are important factors to consider. Providing the best service to the patient, which includes minimizing wait times, should also be considered when designing the process. The steps may vary, but thoughtful planning, with the input from members of the clinical team and patients, creates standard administrative and clinical workflows. Consistent post-encounter processes promote efficiency, enhance the experience of patients and personnel, and reduce the likelihood of errors.

Stage 5: Inter-Encounter

The ambulatory practice plays an important role between F2F encounters with the patient. Unlike other healthcare settings—the hospital, nursing home, and so forth—the patient is not stationary. Servicing the patient, therefore, may require process steps outside of the hallmark encounter between the patient and the clinician. This fifth stage of ambulatory practice operations—the inter-encounter—requires dedicated work processes, tools, resources, and personnel. This section features a review of the following elements of an inter-encounter: care coordination, **care transitions**, communication, and test results.

Care Coordination

Ambulatory practices routinely receive communication from the patient about various aspects of their care between visits. Patients may communicate with the practice about concerns, lifestyle changes, or a host of other issues related to their care. The information conveyed by the patient is incorporated into the patient's record. Additionally, depending on test results, symptoms, medication reactions, and so forth, changes to the care plan may be needed between formal F2F visits, particularly with patients who are managed for chronic illnesses. Personnel assigned to care coordination duties communicate with the patient (or their caregiver). Alterations to the patient's care are documented in the record, as is the details of the conversation with or about the patient.

The inter-encounter work involving care coordination is crucial for an ambulatory practice to consider from a personnel and process perspective. A primary care practice is often referred to as the patient's medical home. The term *home* is indicative of the relationship between the patient and the practice. If the patient feels ill, they may contact the practice for advice and triage; if the patient is due for a preventive service, the practice may communicate a reminder to the patient; and if the patient is discharged from the hospital back to the home for recuperation, the practice may connect with the patient to guide their recovery. A significant body of evidence supports the value of a medical home. Organizations have established credentialing programs for primary care practices such as the NCQA, which recognizes primary care practices that successfully meet the criteria for a patient-centered medical home.

Patients rely on the specialty practice in a similar manner for acute events or chronic conditions. Surgery practices, as well as those practices in which procedures are performed, provide care coordination between visits—for example, connecting with patients about preoperative instructions, postoperative wound care, medication issues, and so forth. Chronic conditions also require inter-encounter management; for example, the caregiver of a patient with Parkinson's may contact a neurology practice for guidance should the patient demonstrate unexpected memory lapses. This may prompt guidance communicated over the phone, or the patient may be scheduled for an appointment.

Care Transitions

Coordination and transitions of care between providers or settings – often collectively called "care transitions"—is a critical inter-encounter task. For example, the practice may receive communication from the hospital regarding all inpatient discharges on the day prior for patients listing the practice as their primary care provider. This communication would prompt personnel at the practice to review the patient's record, incorporate the discharge, and determine the best course of action for transitional care management. Often, this includes proactively calling the patient, checking on the patient's status, and scheduling a hospital follow-up appointment. The ambulatory setting is often the focus of managing patients' care transitions, as it is considered the "hub" of the patient's care among the many "spokes" of the healthcare system. As the ambulatory practice often represents where the patient commences care, the practice manages patients on a longitudinal basis.

Communication

Patients may contact the ambulatory practice, or there may be communication from other clinicians or healthcare personnel, as well as caregivers, partners, and family members about the patient. In a well-managed ambulatory practice, these communications are processed in a timely, consistent manner. The management of communication includes documentation of the receipt of the message, appropriate documentation of the message, and escalation protocols.

A clear, delineated process to manage all inbound and outbound messages, developed with input from all relevant personnel and accompanied by elucidated escalation protocols, should be in place. All messages should be documented, to include the content as well as the timing. The latter is often a function of the practice's EHR system, but there may be various steps that necessitate action to record the timing of tasks. The well-managed practice has an automated procedure for message distribution and resolution; messages that are unattended in a certain time frame—three to a maximum of 24 hours—are routed to a supervisor or manager for immediate attention. A message is not a singular event. Resolving a patient's inquiry may involve a series of follow-up tasks and several communication points. Each of the steps should be documented, to include the final demarcation of completion.

A well-managed ambulatory practice maintains a communication process that promotes patient safety and quality through the construction of streamlined processes for which personnel are held accountable.

Test Results

The ambulatory practice manages a multitude of test results emanating from tests performed at the practice or those which are ordered for tests performed out of the practice. For example, the ambulatory practice may perform complete blood counts (CBC) and urine analyses in an in-house laboratory; patients may be referred to an external facility for a CT scan. Regardless of the location of the test, the process surrounding the receipt, review and action regarding test orders and results is of crucial importance to the well-managed ambulatory practice. According to TJC, "delayed or incomplete test result follow-up, which can lead to missed and/or delayed diagnosis, is an important issue in the ambulatory setting. Delayed test result follow-up has been linked to poorer patient outcomes and increased risk of mortality and accounts for a large portion of medical malpractice claims" (Ai et al., 2018).

The well-managed ambulatory practice designs a process to identify and monitor all test orders and results, as well as the communication to the patient. The process is typically managed via the EHR system. The specifics of the process vary by system; however, the process generally follows a consistent construct of ordering, resulting, and communicating. The clinician orders the test in the system, thereby identifying and associating the test in the patient's record. The test is placed into an open or pending status. When the result is returned, the open or pending order is closed and the result is identified in the system. The EHR system alerts the clinician about the result, often accompanied with a documentation of whether the result falls outside of the normal range and an interpretation of the result. Communication about the results (to include the data) may be transferred to the patient's chart immediately, or the results may be held for a select period (e.g., 24 hours) for the clinician to review prior to the information being released to the patient. The results are posted to the patient portal.

Orders, results, and communication are primarily handled through the EHR system in a well-managed practice. However, there are important considerations related to processes that may fall outside of the automated system. If a test is performed at an external facility, the result may be received outside of the system. This may prompt a conversion to an electronic format, noting that a well-managed ambulatory practice facilitates a comprehensive process for confirming receipt of the result regardless of its entry point. Once received, the practice indexes the result in the appropriate section of the patient's chart. Alternatively, the result may be necessarily managed manually with the data transferred into the patient's record via personnel who transcribe the information. Additionally, critical test results may prompt a call to the practice to precede or accompany the electronic reporting of results. The well-managed ambulatory practice identifies all channels of communication for test ordering, resulting and communication processes to ensure that they are managed effectively and efficiently to support the delivery of safe, quality care.

For many ambulatory practices, both administrative and clinical personnel are tasked with inter-encounter work. Administrative personnel may manage incoming communication to include phone calls, faxes, and portal messages; these personnel may also be involved in outbound communication. For example, a clinician may review a test result, determine that the patient needs to be seen, and, thus, forward a message to the administrative personnel to contact the patient to schedule an appointment. The clinical personnel may handle a significant volume of the activities related to care transition, albeit consulting with the clinician as appropriate. The clinician may then provide advice to the clinical personnel—or assume responsibility for the communication. Regardless of the details of the communication process, escalation protocols are essential.

As discussed earlier in this chapter, escalation protocols involve information that may be communicated by the patient (or the messenger or a caregiver, for example) that indicate a concern that requires immediate attention. For example, if a caregiver calls and reveals that the patient's left arm has gone numb—or their face is drooping, the practice would not take a message but rather act on the situation immediately. The term *escalation* is used because the patient's concern requires rising above the stated process with enhanced attention and associated action.

Some practices have specific personnel designated to inter-encounter tasks; others may assign activities to personnel based on the patient's clinician. As ambulatory practices manage the care of hundreds, perhaps thousands of patients, supportive technology is crucial in ensuring these processes are efficient, as well as comprehensive. The practice's EHR system may facilitate these functions, with the practice opting for an integrated registry or population health management module to assist.

In addition to care coordination, care transitions, communication, and test results, inter-encounter tasks may also include the issuance, renewals or authorizations of prescriptions; disease registry management; notification and assistance with preventive services; insurance referrals and authorization; counseling of caregivers or family members; chronic care management; communication with clinicians or facilities; care transitions; and others.

The volume and variety of inter-encounter tasks performed at an ambulatory practice requires an approach that is supported by technology and involves all associated personnel trained in both process and tools.

TECHNOLOGY

The evolution of technology for the ambulatory practice has been remarkable. The 1980s and 1990s ushered in automation to support business and administrative processes.

These systems, collectively referred to as practice management (PM) systems, introduced technology to manage registration, scheduling, and billing. EHR systems, initially separate from their administrative counterparts, were installed in the 2000s and 2010s. Government funding initiated by the American Recovery and Reinvestment Act spurred the adoption in the 2010s (CMS, 2020). Today, many practices have a single technological solution to manage both the administrative and clinical aspects of the practice; the nomenclature given to these management information systems is the title once reserved for the clinical aspects of the technology—the EHR system.

Electronic Health Record System

According to the federal government (HealthIT.gov, n.d.), "EHRs are . . . digital (computerized) versions of patients' paper charts. EHRs are real-time, patient-centered records. They make information available instantly . . . bring[ing] together in one place everything about a patient's health. EHRs can:

- Contain information about a patient's medical history, diagnoses, medications, immunization dates, allergies, radiology images, and lab and test results;
- Offer access to evidence-based tools that providers can use in making decisions about a patient's care;
- Automate and streamline providers' workflow;
- Increase organization and accuracy of patient information; and
- Support key market changes in payer requirements and consumer expectations."

The introduction of EHR systems in the ambulatory practice demanded significant change in the work processes and workflow of providers and personnel in the ambulatory practice. Their introduction involved a steep learning curve and was not without its challenges. Ambulatory practices also were required to secure information technology support resources via hiring, contracting, or outsourcing to maintain and support hardware, software, and respond to frequently changing regulatory and billing requirements. Today, EHR systems are considered the information highways for an ambulatory practice.

Telemedicine

Telemedicine is the practice of caring for patients in a remote setting with the use of technology. In 1924, the popular magazine *Radio News* featured an image of a patient describing his symptoms to a physician via the radio. Titled *The Radio Doctor – Maybe!* the cartoon was the artist's rendering of a possible future state featuring people talking to a radio with an image of a physician embedded in it. Many years would pass before this vision became reality. There are reports of radiology images being exchanged in the late 1940s (Zundel, 1996) and two-way interactive television in the 1950s (Benschoter, 1967). In 1960, physicians at the National Aeronautics and Space Association used telemedicine to monitor astronauts in flight during the Project Mercury mission (Link, 1965). These pilots led to more activity in the realm of telemedicine, although the expense of the technology and the accompanying transmission of images and data hindered its widespread use into the 1990s (Crump & Pfeil, 1995). As access to affordable, suitable technology increased, the regulations related to performing and being paid for services rendered by telemedicine surged. The Balanced Budget Act of 1997 authorized separate Medicare fee-for-service payment for telehealth as in 1999; however, payments were restricted to limited circumstances (Kasich, 1997). Patients, for example, could not be seen in their homes; furthermore, only patients in designated rural communities would qualify for payment. As a result of these restrictions—and more—imposed in the late 1990s, telemedicine remained at a low utilization through 2020. Only one quarter of a percent (0.25%) of Medicare beneficiaries in the traditional fee-for-service plans used a telehealth service in 2016 (CMS, 2018). Nearly all services in an ambulatory practice were provided on a F2F basis.

The novel coronavirus (COVID-19) pandemic of 2020 ushered in a series of temporary changes related to regulatory relaxation and reimbursement changes, bringing telemedicine into the mainstream of ambulatory care in the United States. During this time, ambulatory practices were required to develop remote work processes for patients with COVID-19 symptoms isolated at home, while managing a full caseload of patients without symptoms in accordance with new safety measures. The pandemic required practices to work diligently and quickly to determine which patients required a F2F visit and which could be safely managed via telemedicine. The operations of an ambulatory practice accommodated the new workflow in rapid order.

The framework for a telemedicine encounter is consistent with that of a F2F visit. It involves each of the five stages of ambulatory practice operations: (1) pre-encounter, (2) arrival, (3) encounter, (4) post-encounter, and (5) inter-encounter. Like F2F visits, patients are registered, scheduled, and arrived prior to their online visit. Patients who have a telemedicine visit may also have tests ordered, follow-up appointments scheduled, and so forth. There are some distinct differences, however, between the workflows for F2F visits and telemedicine visits:

- Pre-Encounter. The pre-encounter functions are performed on a remote basis; this includes obtaining patient signatures on required forms electronically. The responsibilities once performed by front office personnel with the patient physically present are integrated into a pre-encounter process that is performed remotely.

- Clinical Intake. The clinical intake, a component of the patient's arrival, may take place at a different time, thereby bifurcated from the arrival process. The steps involved in telemedicine rooming include ensuring the patient is prepared for the encounter and has the technology enabled in accordance with that which is supported by the vendor's technical specifications; conferring with the patient about the type of data that can be gathered (e.g., does the patient have a blood pressure cuff? a scale? a pulse oximeter?); and obtaining information from the patient and inputting it into the patient's chart for the clinician's review.

The schedule template itself may categorize telemedicine encounters separately from those conducted F2F. This allows the personnel at the practice to appropriately perform and track these encounters. Rather than maintain a separate telemedicine template, many practices have integrated telemedicine and F2F encounters on the same template, although the mechanics of doing so vary by practice. Some have dedicated telemedicine days or sessions; others intersperse the appointments such that each hour has a combination of telemedicine and F2F encounters.

Because the patient is not physically present in the ambulatory practice, the post-encounter management is conducted remotely. The same attention to detail regarding the actions to perform on behalf of the patient is essential for telemedicine encounters.

Personnel, once exclusively dedicated to F2F care, typically manage both F2F and telemedicine encounters. The responsibilities associated with each encounter type should be clearly outlined and assigned to personnel. See the accompanying case study of a company that offers care exclusively via telemedicine, illustrating the changing landscape of ambulatory practice.

PERFORMANCE IMPROVEMENT

The complex, multifaceted operations of an ambulatory practice provide an ideal setting for performance improvement. The approach varies by practice, but two popular improvement methods include **lean production** and systems engineering (see the sidebar "The Importance of Standard Operating Procedures and Metrics" for an ambulatory leader's reflection on key management techniques).

Based on the work of quality guru W. Edwards Deming, the lean production movement got its name from the 1990 book *The Machine That Changed the World: The Story of Lean Production*, authored by researchers at the Massachusetts Institute of Technology. The authors studied the efforts of Toyota to rise to the top of the automobile industry in the 1960s. Their hypothesis was that market changes, increased competition, and a desire to improve profitability helped auto manufacturer Toyota successfully reengineer not only its core processes but also its culture. To make the journey from mass production to lean production, Toyota stripped away—and continues to find and eliminate—waste from the manufacturing process. Instead of relying on inspections of cars after production to determine quality, Toyota integrated

THE IMPORTANCE OF STANDARD OPERATING PROCEDURES AND METRICS

Concettina (Tina) Tolomeo, DNP, MBA, APRN, FNP-BC, AE-C
Senior Director, Patient Access
Yale Medicine
New Haven, Connecticut

The ambulatory healthcare arena is a fast-paced, complex environment. It has become common in recent years for ambulatory practices to merge, making them sizable in both scope and staff. Effective operations, and proper management thereof, serve as the backbone of any successful ambulatory practice. In the ambulatory setting, clinical and administrative staff work together to meet the needs of patients and their families. The ultimate goals of their collaborative efforts are quality patient care that is safe, efficient, and leads to a positive patient experience. To meet these goals, practices must institute two fundamental elements, standard operating procedures (SOPs) and metrics.

Smooth operations don't just happen; they require a plan. W. Edwards Deming, a well-known management consultant, has said, "If you can't describe what you are doing as a process, you don't know what you're doing," thus the importance of SOPs. SOPs set the stage for how a task or process is performed. SOPs aid in training and serve as resources for staff. The belief is that SOPs decrease variation which, in turn, decrease errors and lead to a consistent patient experience. Therefore, SOPs should be established for a variety of patient access and office functions, including, but not limited to, scheduling, check-in, rooming, checkout, and transitions of care.

The model SOP should include the purpose, the specific steps needed to perform the task, a description of documentation required by staff, if any, and outcome measures. Management guru Peter Drucker is often quoted as saying "If you can't measure it, you can't manage it"; hence the importance of including metrics in the SOPs. There are several KPIs that can be used to evaluate the effectiveness of ambulatory SOPs. KPIs in the ambulatory setting include but are not limited to telephony metrics (e.g., abandonment rate, average speed to answer), referral volume, time to schedule new appointments, template utilization, room utilization, and patient satisfaction.

Although vital, it is important to note that establishing SOPs is only the first step. The next step is execution. This step requires clear and effective communication, and often, change management; especially for seasoned staff who do not understand why a new process is necessary because they "have done it this way for years and it works fine." For staff to embrace new workflows, they need to understand and believe in them. This buy-in can be fostered by involving staff in the early stages of SOP development and, by giving them an opportunity to provide feedback.

Once execution has been solidified, it is time to assess the effectiveness of the SOPs. At this stage, it is important to determine if the SOPs are contributing to goal attainment and leading to improvement. This assessment is made by measuring and analyzing the metrics listed in the SOPs. If outcomes are not trending in the right direction, this would be the time to revise the SOPs to improve performance.

Finally, it is important to keep SOPs up to date. System or personnel changes that effect any of the SOP steps must be updated in real time. As previously noted, the ambulatory setting is fast-paced, as a result, the operations must be just as nimble.

quality into the production process. This transformation in thinking, later coined as the Toyota Production System, helped Toyota become the market leader in its industry in terms of sales and market share. How could an ambulatory practice look to an automobile manufacturer's experience to improve its operations?

Two of the original lean production researchers—James P. Womack and Daniel T. Jones—summarized the lean-thinking approach in their 1996 book *Lean Thinking: Banish Waste and Create Wealth in Your Corporation*. The five-step process, which took their teachings about lean production from a manufacturing environment to any industry, espoused:

- Specify value from the customer's perspective.
- Identify all the steps in a process, which collectively is called the "value stream."
- Make the value-creating steps flow toward the customer.
- Let the customer pull value from the next activity.
- Pursue perfection across the organization.

Lean thinking aims to provide the best quality at the lowest cost and in the shortest time through eliminating waste.

A critical step in eliminating waste, and one of the pillars of lean thinking, is formulated by the Five S's. With a goal of minimizing the waste of time, the Five S's represent a visually oriented system for organization the workplace through the following steps:

- Sort: Clear the work area
- Set in order: Designate locations
- Shine: Clean the work area
- Standardize: Everyone doing the same thing, with everything in the same place
- Sustain: Ingrain the process in the organization

To illustrate this tool in an ambulatory practice, let us use the example of a clinical workstation. Consider that a clinical workstation—often referred to as the "nurses' station"—is one of the most visually chaotic areas of a practice. There are computers, phones, note pads, reference books, forms, bins, and lots of sticky notes with instructions. The Five S's tool helps us to (a) sort the tasks and function of the clinical workstation, (b) designate and label everything; (c) keep the workstation clean and orderly, (d) standardize the layout of the tasks and functions; (e) determine a consistent approach and protocol for each task and function, (f) pool the personnel's collective knowledge of the inbound and outbound work and standardize both, and (g) break habits by codifying expectations through personnel engagement, performance evaluations, protocol handbooks, and checklists.

Focusing on a clinical workstation is one of many areas of an ambulatory practice that can benefit from lean. Consider using the "Plan, Do, Check, Act" (PDCA) cycle as the framework for the initiatives. The PDCA cycle has four stages:

Plan: Establish the goal for a process and the steps necessary to achieve it

Do: Implement the proposed changes

Check: Analyze the results in terms of the performance of the process

Act: Based on the results, standardize and stabilize the change by incorporating it in the process

Table 5.4 offers additional lean tools that are commonly applied in ambulatory practices.

TABLE 5.4 Lean Tools for Ambulatory Practice Operations Improvement

VALUE STREAM MAPPING	A detailed visual documentation of a process, to include material and information flow. The improvement process typically starts with a value stream map of the current state and finishes with the future state.
KANBAN	A signal or sign that offers direction to pull work in when—and only when—a resource is needed. Typically organized as visual project management tool, an ambulatory practice may have a "Kanban board" to view its work in progress. This visualization allows observers to identify opportunities for improvement.
KAIZEN	Meaning "change for better," this term refers to events held to improve a system or process to create more value with less waste; typically a multiday event, the key is engaging all personnel to redesign the system or process from the ground up.
POKA YOKE	A term that translates to "mistake proofing," this concept is used to build tools to aid operations. The focus is on improving the process rather than blaming people for errors; examples include requiring a field or value in the EHR system, establishing a container for a supply in which that and only that supply fits, or a checklist accompanied by a picture of a procedure setup.
ISHIKAWA DIAGRAM	A causal diagram, often referred to as a "fishbone diagram" for its shape, the figure documents the potential causes of an event or activity. Named for the Japanese organizational theorist, this cause and cause-and-effect diagram can be used to analyze opportunities to improve performance.

CONCLUSION

Each of the five stages of ambulatory practice operations—(1) pre-encounter, (2) arrival, (3) encounter, (4) post-encounter, and (5) inter-encounter—involve critical clinical and administrative tasks that must be aligned and integrated to ensure patients receive high quality care and service, while maintaining the financial health of the practice. Although the steps associated with a single encounter can be articulated and performed with ease, there are dozens, if not hundreds, of these encounters performed each day, all of which represent varying situations. Supplement these focused activities with the reality of managing patients between and after their encounters, and one can quickly recognize why ambulatory practice operations require special knowledge, attention, and skill.

DISCUSSION QUESTIONS

1. How can a provider ease the stress or worry or simply have good "bedside manner" with a patient during a telemedicine visit?

2. What are some examples of social determinants of health that would be taken into consideration when trying to personalize care for a patient in an ambulatory practice?

3. How might technology be further implemented into the five stages of ambulatory operations without jeopardizing the jobs of clinicians and personnel?

REFERENCES

Ai, A., Desai, S., Shellman, A., & Wright, A. (2018). Understanding test results follow-up in the ambulatory setting: Analysis of multiple perspectives. *The Joint Commission Journal on Quality and Patient Safety, 44*(11), 674–682. https://doi.org/10.1016/j.jcjq.2018.04.011

Benschoter, R. A. (1967). V. Television. Multi-purpose television. *Annals of the New York Academy of Sciences, 142*(2), 471–478. https://doi.org/10.1111/j.1749-6632.1967.tb14360.x

Centers for Medicare and Medicaid Services. (2018, November 15). *Information on Medicare telehealth.* https://www.cms.gov/About-CMS/Agency-Information/OMH/Downloads/Information-on-Medicare-Telehealth-Report.pdf

Centers for Medicare and Medicaid Services. (2020a). *Certified EHR technology.* https://www.cms.gov/Regulations-and-Guidance/Legislation/EHRIncentivePrograms/Certification

Centers for Medicare and Medicaid Services. (2020b). *Medicare program integrity manual: Chapter 3—Verifying potential errors and taking corrective actions.* https://www.cms.gov/Regulations-and-Guidance/Guidance/Manuals/Downloads/pim83c03.pdf

Crump, W. J., & Pfeil, T. A. (1995). Telemedicine primer: An introduction to the technology and an overview of the literature. *Archive of Family Medicine, 4*(9), 796–803. https://doi.org/10.1001/archfami.4.9.796

HealthIT.gov. (n.d.). *Electronic health records: The basics.* https://www.healthit.gov/faq/what-information-does-electronic-health-record-ehr-contain

Institute for Healthcare Improvement. (n.d.). *Huddles.* http://www.ihi.org/resources/Pages/Tools/Huddles.aspx

The Joint Commission. (2020a). *Quick Safety Issue 45: People, processes, health IT and accurate patient identification.* https://www.jointcommission.org/resources/news-and-multimedia/newsletters/newsletters/quick-safety/quick-safety-45-people-processes-health-it-and-accurate-patient-identification/

The Joint Commission. (2020b). *Two patient identifiers—Understanding the requirements.* https://www.jointcommission.org/standards/standard-faqs/home-care/national-patient-safety-goals-npsg/000001545/

Kasich, J. (1997). *H.R.2015 - 105th Congress (1997–1998): Balanced budget act of 1997.* https://www.congress.gov/bill/105th-congress/house-bill/2015

Link, M. M. (1965). *Space medicine in Project Mercury.* (NASA SP-4003, NASA Special Publication). Office of Manned Space Flight, National Aeronautics and Space Administration. https://history.nasa.gov/SP-4003.pdf

Perednia, D. A., & Allen, A. (1995). Telemedicine technology and clinical applications. *Journal of the American Medical Association, 273*(6), 483–487. https://doi.org/10.1001/jama.273.6.483

National Committee for Quality Assurance. (2018). *Guidelines for medical record documentation* https://www.ncqa.org/wp-content/uploads/2018/07/20180110_Guidelines_Medical_Record_Documentation.pdf

UCSF Center for Excellence in Primary Care. (2013). *Healthy huddles.* https://cepc.ucsf.edu/healthy-huddles

Versel, N. (2004). Online reservations: Letting patients make their own appointments. *American Medical News, 22,* 29.

Williams, K. A., Chambers, C. G., Dada, M., McLeod, J. C., & Ulatowski, J. A. (2014). Patient punctuality and clinic performance: Observations from an academic-based private practice pain centre: A prospective quality improvement study. *BMJ Open, 4,* e004679. https://doi.org/10.1136/bmjopen-2013-004679

Womack, J. P., & Jones, D. T. (1996). *Lean thinking: Banish waste and create wealth in your corporation.* Simon and Schuster.

Woodcock, E., Nokes, D., Bolton, H., Bartholomew, D. B. S., Johnson, E., & Shakarchi, A. F. (2020, July/September). The influence of the scheduling horizon on new patient arrivals. *Journal of Ambulatory Care Management, 43*(3), 221–229. https://doi.org/10.1097/JAC.0000000000000334

Yu, E. (2015). *Daily team huddles.* Team-based Learning.

Zundel, K. M. (1996). Telemedicine: History, applications, and impact on librarianship. *Bulletin of the Medical Library Association, 84*(1), 71–79. https://www.ncbi.nlm.nih.gov/pmc/articles/PMC226126/

Case Study

Lemonaid Health: Pursuing a New Strategy in Mental Health

Dr. Davis Liu, cief clinical officer of Lemonaid Health, hung up the phone. The call had been from the company's head of operations based in San Francisco, reporting average turnaround times for provider consultation videos had doubled from 15 minutes to nearly 30 in the last month. This call was accompanied by several emails from physicians and providers expressing frustration about increased workload. Still well within the range of the guaranteed 24-business-hour turnaround, the information had piqued his interest as he knew that speed was crucial to maintain Lemonaid's top-rated net promoter score of 89. "Super-fast" is how the turnaround time is described to potential customers online, and that is what he intended to deliver.

So what was happening? He opened the spreadsheet that showed the volumes of encounters and started drilling into the data. Visits had surged in the first quarter (Q1) of 2020 in light of the COVID-19 pandemic; the greatest increase was due to encounters related to depression and anxiety. Mental health visits and medications for this new line of business—launched in May 2019—had increased dramatically. The recurring revenue model—$95 per month, in addition to a decent margin on medications that may be prescribed—was adding needed cash to the company's bottom line. Management and investors were enthused about the performance of this new line of business. However, did the doubling of turnaround times portend a problem? Or, was Lemonaid on the edge of an incredible opportunity—the mental health market—that simply needed to be better resourced?

How Lemonaid Works

Under the tagline *"Great Care You Can Afford,"* Lemonaid Health offers convenient, accessible, and affordable medical care through an asynchronous telemedicine platform (the company's mission is presented in Box 5.1). Consumers receive virtual consultations with a licensed healthcare provider for a variety of low-acuity needs. As clinically appropriate, medications are prescribed and mailed directly to the consumer via Lemonaid's pharmacy.

Amy Shim, Rollins School of Public Health'21; Christina Aaron, Duke University'25; and Jacqueline Hackett and Robert Kononowech, DrPH students, JHSPH, contributed to the case study. The support of Dr. Davis Liu and Lemonaid Health was invaluable to creating this case study. More information about Lemonaid Health can be found at: www.lemonaidhealth.com

BOX 5.1   LEMONAID HEALTH'S MISSION

Our mission is to bring ultra low cost healthcare to everyone in America. We want to make primary care so affordable and accessible that everyone can get great care when they need it, regardless of insurance.

SOURCE: *Our mission.* https://www.lemonaidhealth.com/our-mission

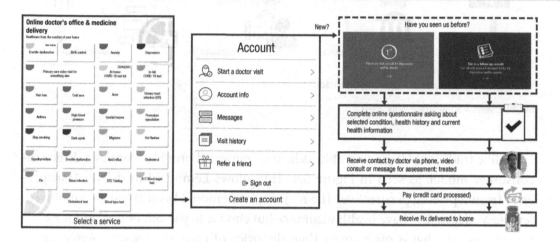

FIGURE 5.3 Patient flow at Lemonaid.

SOURCE: Original to Lemonaid, June 2020. Reprinted by permission.

Lemonaid offers several dozen services, including primary care, sexual healthcare, hair-loss treatment, erectile dysfunction treatment, chronic condition care, psychiatric care, a COVID-19 antibody test, and more. A customer may also request a primary care video visit for an issue not already listed on its website or smartphone app.

In the typical Lemonaid scenario, a patient launches the Lemonaid Health platform online or via an app; the patient selects a service from a listing of services offered and subsequently completes a set of health questions. A credit card is entered at the conclusion of this stage for payment related to the consultation – visits start at $25 for most services; no health insurance is accepted.

On the back end, the responses are reviewed by a Lemonaid physician or advanced practice provider (APP), who may video call the patient, call a patient by phone, and/ or send a secure message to communicate with the patient. After assessing the patient's condition and appropriateness for treatment, a plan is created and communicated to the patient. The physician or APP may write a prescription for the patient based on their diagnosis; the patient's credit card is charged, and a prescription is sent, by mail, to the address designated by the customer by Lemonaid's pharmacy (patient flow is shown in Figure 5.3). When a patient's symptoms do not fit one of the conditions Lemonaid diagnoses or there are other issues of concern noted by Lemonaid's clinical team, the physician or APP may advise the patient to visit a doctor in person and refund the consultation fee.

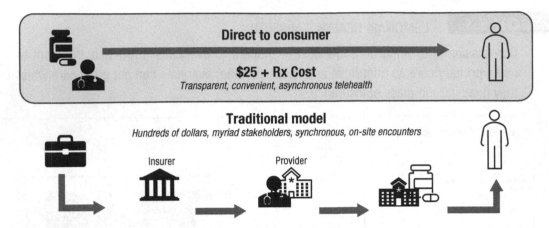

FIGURE 5.4 Lemonaid's business model.

SOURCE: Author's rendering. May 2020.

Unlike traditional financing of healthcare, Lemonaid provides care in a direct-to-consumer model, as seen in Figure 5.4. This allows Lemonaid to deliver transparency from a pricing perspective. The majority of Lemonaid's customers—employed, female Millennials—have health insurance but choose to pay out of pocket for a convenient service that is often lower than the price of their copayment. Avoiding an embarrassing F2F interaction with a physician is also cited as a primary reason for using Lemonaid, according to company research.

Physically situated at their San Francisco headquarters, Lemonaid's three physicians are licensed to provide services in all 50 states and Washington D.C., one of only a handful of telemedicine services licensed to operate nationwide. State-by-state regulations and licensure make it costly and difficult to open in a new state, thereby making Lemonaid's regulatory compliance an advantage.

Lemonaid owns its infrastructure, including its technology stack and pharmacy. The technology system features a sophisticated platform for communicating with the patient during and after an encounter. The pharmacy is situated in the Midwest, mailing prescriptions throughout the United States. The company purchases the prescriptions from a group purchasing organization, which buys the medications from the manufacturers. Only a limited number of medications are dispensed and distributed; most are available as low-cost generic drugs. Like the consultation, patients pay directly for their medications, so they must be priced competitively.

Unlike many of its competitors, Lemonaid employs its own physicians and advanced practice providers. The ability to control quality from an administrative and clinical perspective is perceived as critical to the business' success, specifically the ability to provide a seamless user experience at every touch point and deliver high-quality medical care. Custom, evidence-based protocols drive every encounter, so quality can be managed centrally and in real time. On the flip side, the infrastructure is costly.

Commencing operations in 2014, Lemonaid has developed an impeccable reputation (A+ BBB [Better Business Bureau] rating), high customer satisfaction (4.9/5 rating on the Apple App store), and high employee satisfaction (4.7/5 on Glassdoor).

After the COVID-19 pandemic hit in Q1 2020, Lemonaid partnered with Quest Diagnostics to provide a COVID-19 antibody test as an addition to their existing services. Customers would visit a Quest Diagnostics lab to take the test and receive their results via their Lemonaid account. Lemonaid also has a pending partnership with Scanwell Health to provide at-home COVID-19 antibody tests. The in-lab antibody test is available; the at-home antibody test is pending U.S. Food and Drug Administration (FDA) approval.

Telemedicine Market

Pre-pandemic predictions of the telemedicine market were projected to be a $35 billion market by 2025 (Table 5.5). However, as a result of the pandemic, estimates of telemedicine growth have been expected to increase. A 2020 McKinsey report indicates that 20% of all U.S. healthcare spending—approximately $250 million—could be administered virtually, including nearly a quarter of all office visits (Bestsennyy et al., 2020).

Consumer Demand. A multitude of factors contribute to the growth of the telemedicine market. Consumer expectations are shifting: 60% of participants in a recent survey reported that they would "absolutely" or would be "very likely" to change healthcare providers if the new provider offered "an experience that includes

TABLE 5.5 Total U.S. Telemedicine Market Size Forecast 2014–2025 (in billions)

YEAR	MARKET SIZE ($)
2014	6.1
2015	7.2
2016	8.4
2017	10
2018	11.5
2019	13.5
2020	15.9
2021	18.7
2022	22
2023	25.5
2024	29.8
2025	35

SOURCE: Adapted from Statista (2018, November). *Grand view research ID938551.*

faster appointments, online booking and video appointments" (econsultancy, 2019). An American Hospital Association study indicates that "70% of U.S. patients are comfortable communicating with their healthcare professionals over text, email, or video" (BCC Research Staff, 2018). For younger generations, telemedicine is particularly well-suited; a recent survey reveals that the generation of Millennials do not desire human contact when purchasing a product or service (ABBYY, 2018).

With employer-sponsored health insurance plans shifting toward higher deductibles, consumers are increasingly empowered in their choice of healthcare spending (Hamel et al., 2019; Healthcare Global, 2015). The cost of a virtual consultation by Lemonaid, typically starting at $25, is comparable or less than a patient copay cost through many health insurance companies. Receiving direct services from Lemonaid also eliminates the hassle of having to shop around for a provider who is taking new patients or is in-network with their insurance company. Consumers are attracted—and empowered— by the information symmetry made possible by Lemonaid's price transparency.

The direct-to-consumer model is not the only means to address consumer demand for telemedicine. Many telemedicine companies contract with insurance providers to integrate into their array of services. Telemedicine offerings have grown tremendously over the years. As of 2019, approximately 90% of large U.S. employer-based health insurance plans offered telemedicine services, as shown in Figure 5.5.

The COVID-19 pandemic may permanently change the demand for telemedicine services. Many consumers were interested in the past, but the pandemic has accelerated consumer demand. Not only were many physician's offices closed and patients fearful of being exposed to COVID-19 through an in-person office visit, but the economic situation also drove consumers to seek low-cost, transparent pricing options for care. Outpatient visits plummeted nearly 60% from the first week of March 2020 to the last (Figure 5.6), according to a study published by the Commonwealth Fund led by Harvard University researchers (Mehrotra et al., 2020). Insurance payers expanded coverage of telemedicine visits in March to meet a growing demand for care outside of the traditional physical encounter with a physician; the passage of the Families First Coronavirus Response Act in April 2020 required coverage for COVID-19 testing and related encounters—in person *or* telemedicine—in full by all private and public insurance payers. Blue Cross Blue Shield of Tennessee was among the first payers to announce that coverage of telemedicine would be permanent (Blue Cross Blue Shield of Tennessee, n.d.).

Some payers—such as Humana—are partnering with suppliers to offer telemedicine directly to their beneficiaries. Humana has partnered with telemedicine provider Doctor on Demand, while United Healthcare, Aetna, and many other commercial insurers are pitching members access to telemedicine at no cost. As in the example, these services are typically provided to consumers who are enrolled in the insurance product at no cost.

Provider Supply. Telemedicine platforms are readily available to physicians and advanced practice providers, with hundreds of companies from which to choose. Significant investments have been put into computerized records and patient communication

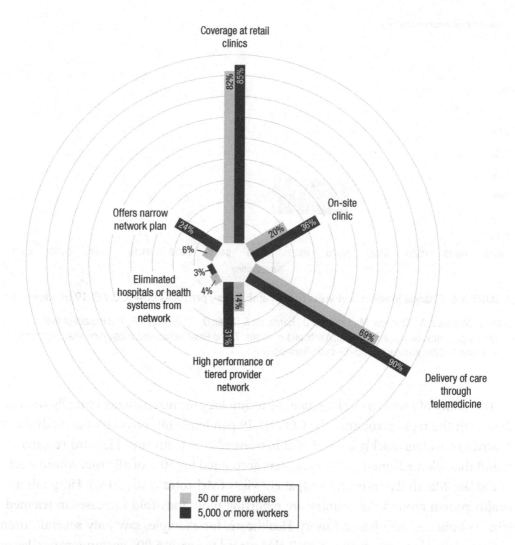

FIGURE 5.5 Features of health plans by firm size, 2019.

NOTE: For retail clinics, telemedicine, and high performance/tiered provider network, firms were asked if their plan with the largest enrollment had these features.

SOURCE: Data from KFF. (2020, October 8). *Kaiser Family Foundation's employer health benefits survey 2019.* https://www.kff.org/health-costs/report/2020-employer-health-benefits-survey/

platforms, due to the Obama administration's EHR Incentive Program (Centers for Medicare and Medicaid Services [CMS], n.d.-b). As of 2017, nearly nine in 10 office-based physicians had adopted an EHR system (Office of the National Coordinator for Healthcare Information Technology, n.d.). Despite the availability of technology, however, providers' adoption rate remained fairly low—annual telemedicine visits evaluated from a large insurers' claims database showed just 6.57 telemedicine encounters per 1,000 members in 2017, with the majority being mental health (53%; Barnett et al., 2018). Despite the overall technology adoption by U.S. physicians in the past decade, telemedicine take-up rates have been slow, largely due to regulatory and reimbursement issues.

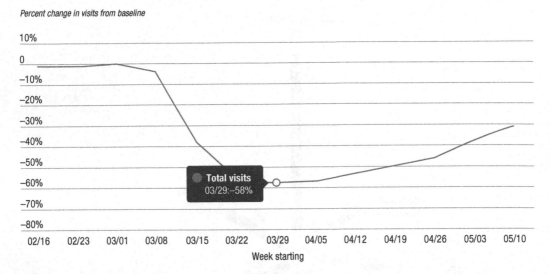

FIGURE 5.6 Change in volume of visits to U.S. ambulatory practices after COVID-19 pandemic hit.

SOURCE: Mehrotra, A., Chernew, M., Linetsky, D., Hatch, H., & Cutler, D. (2020, May 19). The impact of the COVID-19 pandemic on outpatient visits: A rebound emerges. *To the Point.* https://www.commonwealthfund.org/publications/2020/apr/impact-covid-19-outpatient-visits

The ability of providers to integrate the technology to treat patients virtually was evident with the rapid pivot after the COVID-19 pandemic hit; physicians and advanced practice providers quickly transitioned to telemedicine platforms. Harvard researchers found that telemedicine-based encounters accounted for 30% of all visits within weeks of the late-March dip in overall outpatient visits (Mehrotra et al., 2020). Hospitals and health system around the country are reporting thousands-fold increases in telemedicine volume; Atlanta-based Emory Healthcare, for example, saw only several dozen patients daily via telemedicine in 2019; this surged to nearly 6,000 encounters per day in May 2020 (Kier, 2020).

Public and private companies have flocked to meet the surging consumer demand resulting from the pandemic. The projected five-year journey for on-demand virtual visits was transformed to a fraction of the time as the COVID-19 pandemic has catalyzed the movement towards these services.

Yet providers may not be able to keep pace with demand. For example, the publicly traded telemedicine company Teladoc announced a 50% increase in services demanded between the week of March 13, 2020, and the week of March 20, 2020, but customers also reported significantly longer wait times for appointments and even cancellations after waiting extended periods of time for service (Olson, 2020).

In addition to telemedicine, mail-order prescriptions businesses have proliferated, growing 21% between 2019 and 2020 and holding 5.8% of the prescription drug market share (Hopkins, 2020). Pharmacies across the United States are offering or arranging free delivery services to patients' homes (Olson, 2020).

Regulatory and Reimbursement Environment

Inconsistent, state-based licensing and challenging reimbursement policies complicate the telemedicine industry. State-by-state regulations exist for telemedicine, making operations nationwide a tricky process.

Regulations—including the challenging state licensure issues—crumbled after a public health emergency was declared for the COVID-19 pandemic. On March 13, 2020, the requirement for physicians to hold a license in the state in which services are rendered was temporarily waived by the federal government (Public Health Emergency, n.d.). Such barriers to telemedicine, as detailed in Figure 5.7, were waived temporarily due to the pandemic.

Before the rules were suspended, physicians had to be registered to practice in the state in which the patient resides. To further complicate the process, each state has its own procedure and laws for licensing (BCC Research Staff, 2018). Telehealth providers also have to consider liability insurance, in which some liability insurance only covers encounters administered in the state that the physician resides (BCC Research Staff, 2018). Steps are needed to adhere to the federal law designed to protect patients' privacy, as an increased threat of putting patients' medical information at risk exists (Center for Internet Security, n.d.).

Medications are also highly regulated, particularly those that are provided by mail. As the opioid crisis deepened, the federal government cracked down on many fraudulent online pharmacies (FDA, n.d.). Pharmacies are subject to a host of issues, to include licensing and inspections that are controlled at the state level (National Association of Boards of Pharmacy, n.d.). State policies also regulate who can prescribe

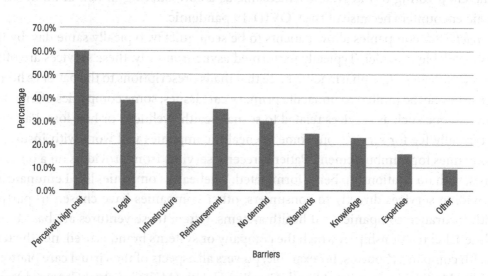

FIGURE 5.7 Barriers to telemedicine.

SOURCE: Courtesy BCC Research. World Health Organization as cited by BCC Research Staff. (2018, June). *Global markets for telemedicine technologies* (BCC Research. Report #HLC014J).

what kind of medication under whose supervision. Like physician licensure, all of this is regulated by each state, with no consistency. Navigating compliance is challenging—and costly.

Reimbursement for telemedicine also varies by state. Many states have parity laws for private insurance, so telehealth visits must be reimbursed as an equivalent in-person visit would be (Center for Connected Health Policy, n.d.). However, payers may limit access to coverage for telemedicine; some health plans cover telemedicine for their beneficiaries, and others do not. The same inconsistency in policy applies to mental health; despite a federal law requiring parity, health insurers have varying protocols related to coverage, claiming that some services are not medically necessary (Graham, 2013). Regardless of the clinical condition, Medicare covers asynchronous telehealth only in rare circumstances, and limits synchronous coverage to patients who are geographically situated in a health professional shortage area (HPSA; CMS, n.d.-c).

Competitive Landscape

The growing market for non-face-to-face care creates a more competitive environment for telemedicine. With the near elimination of regulations related to telemedicine that resulted from the pandemic, public and private companies have flocked to meet the surging consumer demand. As seen in Table 5.6, there are myriad companies like Lemonaid, although they may specialize in specific services, target different customer segments, outsource key infrastructure elements, or require insurance. Lemonaid competes with companies offering telemedicine, as well as virtual primary care and direct primary care. Along with other companies providing non-face-to-face care, Lemonaid now also must compete with traditional healthcare systems and retailers pivoting to integrate telemedicine as a core offering in lieu of ambulatory clinic encounters because of the COVID-19 pandemic.

Telehealth companies allow patients to be seen quickly, typically same day, by the first available provider. Typically performed asynchronously, these services are often paired with an online pharmacy service that mails prescriptions to the patient's home. Services may be limited to nonacute primary care issues; some companies offer a narrower scope such as services related to sexual health, wellness, or hair loss. Payment is typically fee for service, but some telehealth companies will work with insurance companies for reimbursement. Patients receive services from providers on a onetime basis, with no relationship being formulated. Telehealth companies like Lemonaid are providing services directly to consumers; other companies have chosen to partner with insurance companies and health systems. Often, these ventures are based on a white-label relationship in which the company or system's brand is used, not the telehealth company. Zipnosis, for example, powers all aspects of the virtual care platform for the Medical University of South Carolina Health (MUSC Virtual Care, n.d.).

Virtual primary care is a modality in which traditional hospitals and health systems, physician practices, or individual clinicians offer primary care services via

TABLE 5.6 Lemonaid's Market Competitors

COMPANY	WEBSITE	MODEL	SERVICE OFFERINGS	TARGET DEMO-GRAPHIC	PRICING INFO	NOTES
HIMS & HERS	https://www.forhims.com/ https://www.forhers.com/	Teleheath (specialty focus)	Hair Loss/Care, Sexual Health, Skin Care, Mental Health, General Primary Care, Supplements	Hims: for men Hers: for women	Free initial consultations for many conditions, $39 for primary care visit	Now offering primary care visits, own product lines and kit sets, COVID-19 lab test, mental health (anonymous support groups, individual therapy and psychiatry/medication coming soon)
RO (INCLUDES ROMAN, RORY, AND ZERO)	https://www.getroman.com/ https://www.hellorory.com/ https://quitwithzero.com/	Telehealth (specialty focus)	Roman: sexual health, hair and skin, daily health Rory: skin and eyelashes, sexual health, daily health, menopause Zero: smoking cessation	Roman: for Men Rory: for women Zero: for smokers trying to quit	$15 online consultations + Rx costs	Only available in states where Ro has licensed physicians on its platform, custom treatment, and customized products
NURX	https://www.nurx.com/	Telehealth (specialty focus)	Sexual health (birth control, STI testing, emergency contraception)	Women	$15 consultation fee + Various prices for Tests; $5 per month for Rx	Accepts insurance, including Medicaid in some states. Only available in states (@30) where Nurx has licensed physicians and can ship Rx/test kits.

(continued)

TABLE 5.6 Lemonaid's Market Competitors (Continued)

COMPANY	WEBSITE	MODEL	SERVICE OFFERINGS	TARGET DEMO-GRAPHIC	PRICING INFO	NOTES
Doctor on Demand	https://www.doctorondemand.com/	Telehealth	Urgent care, behavioral health, preventive health, chronic care (asthma, weight management, blood pressure, cholesterol, etc.)	Everyone, including children	Pricing depends on your insurance plan and/or employer	Contracts with employers and insurance companies to offer discounted or in-network services to their employers or members. Also serves those who are uninsured
Plush Care	https://plushcare.com/	Direct primary care	Urgent care, behavioral health, preventive health, chronic care, sexual health and wellness, hair loss	Adults	Membership of $14.99 a month, $99 first visit (uninsured), copay for first visit (insured)	Contracts with insurance companies to offer in-network services to their members. Direct primary care model.
MDLive	https://www.mdlive.com/	Telehealth	Urgent care, behavioral health, dermatology	Adults	Varies based on your health plan and the specific condition you wish to consult about	COVID-19 risk assessment but no test
Babylon Health	https://www.babylonhealth.com/us/	Telehealth	Comprehensive primary care	Adults	Co-pay for virtual consultations varies by health insurance provider. Chatbox and HealthCheck features available for free regardless of insurance coverage.	App only. U.K. company (has other locations) expanding into the U.S. market. COVID-19 info but no test

(continued)

TABLE 5.6 Lemonaid's Market Competitors *(Continued)*

COMPANY	WEBSITE	MODEL	SERVICE OFFERINGS	TARGET DEMO-GRAPHIC	PRICING INFO	NOTES
Teladoc Health	https://teladochealth.com/	Telehealth	Comprehensive primary care	Everyone, including children	Available for those whose insurers or health plans offer this in-service. $49 copay for everyday care, more for certain specialty services	One of the first and largest Telehealth companies in the United States, trades on the NYSE, over 27 million members globally. Also offers telehealth software platform for healthcareorganizations
eVisit	https://evisit.com/	Software platform for providers	Telehealth software platform for health care systems, hospitals, providers, etc.	Health Care Providers		VirtualED specifically for COVID-19 response
HealthTap	https://www.healthtap.com/	Direct primary care	Comprehensive primary care	Adults	$10/month membership	Contracts with employers and groups to provide services to their employees/members. Direct primary care model. Does serve individual clients but far less common

SOURCE: Authors; listing not intended to be comprehensive but rather to provide examples of competitors and their offerings. Research conducted in June 2020.

telemedicine utilizing their existing infrastructure. Although such practices can be entirely virtual, often they are an extension of traditional physical in-person practices and thus usually allow the patient to experience a combination of in-person and telehealth services from the same provider(s). Patients typically can be followed by the same provider over time. Reimbursement may be possible through the patient's health plan or directly from the patient; payer–provider organizations like Kaiser Permanente operate under this model.

Direct primary care is a capitated arrangement for primary care in which the health plan, employer, or patient pays a fee per member per month to the primary care provider for access to a broad range of primary care and related administrative services. This delivery model typically offers convenient, 24/7 access through office visits and telemedicine, as well as a bidirectional virtual communication platform. Like virtual primary care, the provider–patient relationship is a hallmark of this model; coordination of care, referrals, and communication are included.

Traditional brick-and-mortar healthcare facilities also compete in this space. Hospitals and physician practices are offering new models of delivery, like the CMS's 2021 launch *Primary Care First* program that demonstrates a departure from the traditional fee-for-service model (CMS, n.d.-a). A growing number of new retail healthcare offerings such as CVS's Health Hub and WalmartHealth create convenient treatment services for primary care conditions, including chronic illness treatment and management.

Mental Health in Telemedicine

Mental health is particularly well-suited to a telemedicine platform due to several inherent factors: high patient demand; acute shortages of qualified providers; the relatively reduced need for laboratory tests, imaging studies, and physical examinations; and the stigma attached to mental illness (Corrigan et al., 2014). Mental health places a significant burden on society in terms of cost, quality of life, morbidity, and mortality. It is estimated that 70% of Americans experience an unmet mental health need (Henderson et al., 2013).

Interest in mental health technologies has existed for several years; a 2015 national survey found mental health applications to be among the top three categories of downloaded health apps (Powell et al., 2019). Telemedicine can improve access to mental care by removing geographical constraints, including expanding services to rural areas where mental health providers are sparse. Multiple barriers to mental health treatment are aggravated by a lack of mental health specialists; consequently, mental health services via telemedicine is useful in meeting the gap in treatment needs (Mohr et al., 2017).

The "dose-dependent" nature of mental healthcare typically equates to long-term follow-up and coordinated care. Telemedicine is often a bridge for in-person services.

Many mental health apps include screenings that encourage people to seek local services; therefore, in-person services may also see a rise in demand (Powell et al., 2019). Researchers Shah et al. (2018) found that virtual visits increased total visits (i.e., virtual plus in-person visits) by 80% over 1.5 years.

The COVID-19 pandemic has brought forth economic distress, significant lifestyle changes or disruptions, and an extended period of uncertainty among many Americans. According to the Kaiser Family Foundation, four in 10 adults reported anxiety-related or depressive symptoms during the pandemic, a high spike from one in 10 adults in the first half of 2019 (Panchal et al., 2021). The pandemic propelled mental health into the spotlight, with experts citing the need for mental health resources to be ramped up for access immediately, as well as an infrastructure to serve the long-term implications associated with the pandemic (Galea et al., 2020). Citing the challenges of COVID-related psychological distress, the international community is calling for a significant investment in mental health services worldwide (United Nations, 2020). "The scaling-up and reorganization of mental health services that is now needed on a global scale is an opportunity to build a mental health system that is fit for the future," said Dévora Kestel, Director of the Department of Mental Health and Substance Use at the World Health Organization (2020, "An Opportunity"). The infrastructure for mental health services in the United States is not well positioned for this growing demand, as highlighted in Figure 5.8. Sixty-five percent of nonmetropolitan U.S. counties do not have a psychiatrist, and nearly half of nonmetropolitan counties have no psychologist (Andrilla et al., 2018).

The Decision Looms

Dr. Liu had to decide swiftly, as it would take several months to recruit and on-board providers to handle the mental health offerings. Should Lemonaid Health embrace the growing mental health business? Is this line of business consistent with the company's strategy? Why or why not?

Questions to Consider (with accompanying reading)

1. Reading: Treacy, M., & Wiersema, F. (1993). Customer intimacy and other value disciplines. *Harvard Business Review, 71*(1), 84–93.

According to Treacy and Wiersema, operational excellence means companies provide "customers with reliable products or services at competitive prices and delivered with minimal difficulty or inconvenience"; customer intimacy means companies "continually tailor and shape products and services to fit an increasingly fine definition of the customer"; and product leadership means companies "strive to produce a continuous stream of state-of-the-art products and services." Which of Treacy and Wiersema's value discipline does Lemonaid represent: operational excellence, customer intimacy, or product leadership? If Dr. Liu decides to expand the mental

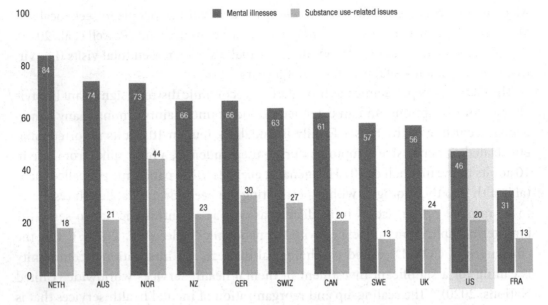

FIGURE 5.8 Primary care practice preparedness to manage patients with mental illnesses or substance-abuse related disorders, 2019.

NOTE: Reflects primary care physicians who reported that their practices are "well prepared," with respect to having sufficient skills and experience, to manage care for patients with mental illnesses (e.g., anxiety, mild or moderate depression) or substance use–related issues (e.g., drug, opioid, alcohol use).

*Other response categories: "somewhat prepared," "not prepared." Data exclude those who said "do not see these patients" (0–2% for mental illness; <1%–10% for substance use–related issues).

DATA: 2019 Commonwealth Fund International Health Policy Survey of Primary Care Physicians.

SOURCE: Tikkanen, R., Fields, K., Williams, R. D., II, & Abrams, M. K. (2020, May 21). *Mental health conditions and substance use: Comparing U.S. needs and treatment capacity with those in other high-income countries.* The Commonwealth Fund. https://www.commonwealthfund.org/publications/issue-briefs/2020/may/mental-health-conditions-substance-use-comparing-us-other-countries

health offering, would this represent a decision consistent with the company's value discipline? Why or why not?

2. Reading: Drucker, P. F. (1994). The theory of the business (cover story). *Harvard Business Review, 72*(5), 95–104.

In *The Theory of the Business*, Peter Drucker describes the importance of understanding an organization's strategic intent. Would Lemonaid's shift to mental health represent a change in the company's "theory of business," according to Peter Drucker? Why or why not?

3. Reading: Porter, M. E. (1998). *Competitive strategy: Techniques for analyzing industries and competitors.* Free Press.

What is Lemonaid's generic strategy, according to Michael Porter: overall cost leadership, differentiation, or focus? Alternatively, is Lemonaid "stuck in the middle"?

4. Reading: Porter, M. (1979, May). How competitive forces shape strategy. *Harvard Business Review, 57*(2), 137–145. https://doi.org/10.1007/978-1 -349-20317-8_10

Examine the threat level of each of Michael Porter's Five Forces (suppliers, buyers, competitive force, new entrants, and substitutes); which forces have a high threat level, and which are low? Justify each response.

REFERENCES FOR CASE STUDY

ABBYY. (2018, June). *Generational divide as millennials look to avoid human interaction.* https://www.abbyy.com/en-us/news/generational-divide-as-millenials-look-to-avoid-human -interaction/#sthash.uPZiJev1.dpbs

Andrilla, H. A., Patterson, D. G., Garberson, L. A., Coulthard, C., & Larson, E. H. (2018, June 1). Geographic variation in the supply of selected behavioral health providers. *American Journal of Preventive Medicine, 54*(6, Suppl. 3), S199–S207. https://www.ajpmonline.org/article/S0749 -3797(18)30005-9/fulltext

Barnett, M., Ray, K., Souza, J., & Mehrotra, A. (2018). Trends in telemedicine use in a large commercially insured population, 2005–2017. *JAMA, 320*(20), 2147–2149. https://jamanetwork .com/journals/jama/fullarticle/2716547

BCC Research Staff. (2018, June). *Global markets for telemedicine technologies* (Report #HLC014J). BCC Research.

Bestsennyy, O., Gilbert, G., Harris, A., & Rost, J. (2020, May 29). *Telehealth: A quarter-trillion -dollar post-COVID-19 reality?* McKinsey & Company Our Insights. https://www.mckinsey .com/industries/healthcare-systems-and-services/our-insights/telehealth-a-quarter-trillion -dollar-post-covid-19-reality#

Blue Cross Blue Shield of Tennessee. (n.d.). *Press release: BlueCross making in-network telehealth services permanent.* BCBST News. https://bcbstnews.com/pressreleases/bluecross-making-in -network-telehealth-services-permanent/

Center for Connected Health Policy. (n.d.). https://www.cchpca.org/all-telehealth-policies/

Center for Internet Security. (n.d.). *Homepage.* https://www.cisecurity.org/

Centers for Medicare and Medicaid Services. (n.d.-a). *Primary care first model options.* https:// innovation.cms.gov/innovation-models/primary-care-first-model-options

Centers for Medicare and Medicaid Services. (n.d.-b). *Promoting interoperability programs.* https:// www.cms.gov/Regulations-and-Guidance/Legislation/EHRIncentivePrograms

Centers for Medicare and Medicaid Services. (n.d.-c) *Telehealth.* https://www.medicare.gov/ coverage/telehealth

The consumerism of healthcare. (2019, February). https://www.adobe.com/content/dam/acom/en/indu stries/healthcare/pdfs/adobe-econsultancy-2019-report-the-consumerization-of-healthcare.pdf

Corrigan, P. W., Druss, B. G., & Perlick, D. A. (2014). The impact of mental illness stigma on seeking and participating in mental health care. *Psychological Science in the Public Interest, 1*(10), 37–70. https://doi.org/10.1177/1529100614531398

econsultancy, with Adobe. (2019, February). *The consumerism of healthcare.* https://www.adobe .com/content/dam/acom/en/industries/healthcare/pdfs/adobe-econsultancy-2019-report-the -consumerization-of-healthcare.pdf

Families First Coronavirus Response Act and Coronavirus Aid, Relief, and Economic Security Act. (2020). https://www.cms.gov/files/document/FFCRA-Part-42-FAQs.pdf

Galea, S., Merchant, R. M., & Lurie, N. (2020). The mental health consequences of COVID-19 and physical distancing: The need for prevention and early intervention. *JAMA Internal Medicine, 180*(6), 817–818. https://doi.org/10.1001/jamainternmed.2020.1562

Graham, J. (2013, March 11). Since 2008, insurers have been required by law to cover mental health—Why many still don't. *The Atlantic.* https://www.theatlantic.com/health/archive/2013/03/since-2008-insurers-have-been-required-by-law-to-cover-mental-health-why-many-still-dont/273562/

Hamel, L., Muñana, C., & Brodie, M. (2019). *Kaiser Family Foundation/LA times survey of adults with employer-sponsored health insurance.* http://files.kff.org/attachment/Report-KFF-LA-Times-Survey-of-Adults-with-Employer-Sponsored-Health-Insurance

Healthcare Global. (2015). *The uber-fication of health care: From a business to consumer model.* https://www.healthcareglobal.com/technology/uber-fication-health-care-business-consumer-model

Henderson, C., Evans-lacko, S., & Thornicroft, G. (2013). Mental illness stigma, help seeking, and public health programs. *American Journal of Public Health, 103*(5), 777–780. https://doi.org/10.2105/AJPH.2012.301056

Hopkins, J. (2020, May 12). Mail-order drug delivery rises during coronavirus lockdowns. *Wall Street Journal.* https://www.wsj.com/articles/mail-order-drug-delivery-rises-during-coronavirus-lockdowns-11589281203

Kier, S. (2020). *Emory healthcare.* Personal correspondence with Author on May 27, 2020.

Mehrotra, A., Chernew, M., Linetsky, D., Hatch, H., & Cutler, D. (2020, May 19). The impact of the COVID-19 pandemic on outpatient visits: A rebound emerges. *To the Point..* https://www.commonwealthfund.org/publications/2020/apr/impact-covid-19-outpatient-visits

Mohr, D. C., Lyon, A. R., Lattie, E. G, Reddy, M., & Schueller, S. M. (2017). Accelerating digital mental health research from early design and creation to successful implementation and sustainment. *Journal of Medical Internet Research, 19*(5), e153. https://doi.org/10.2196/jmir.7725

MUSC Virtual Care. (n.d.). *Homepage.* https://muscvirtualcare.zipnosis.com/

National Association of Boards of Pharmacy. (n.d.). *Verified pharmacy program.* https://nabp.pharmacy/programs/verified-pharmacy-program/

Office of the National Coordinator for Healthcare Information Technology. (n.d.). *Percentage of office-based physicians using any electronic health record (EHR)/electronic medical record (EMR) system and physicians that have a certified EHR/EMR system, by U.S. state: National Electronic Health Records Survey, 2017.* https://dashboard.healthit.gov/quickstats/pages/physician-ehr-adoption-trends.php

Olson, P. (2020, April 1). Telemedicine, once a hard sell, can't keep up with demand. *Wall Street Journal.* https://www.wsj.com/articles/telemedicine-once-a-hard-sell-cant-keep-up-with-demand-11585734425

Panchal, N., Kamal, R., Cox, C., & Garfield, R. (2021, February 10). The implications of COVID-19 for mental health and substance use. *Kaiser Family Foundation.* https://www.kff.org/coronavirus-covid-19/issue-brief/the-implications-of-covid-19-for-mental-health-and-substance-use/

Powell, A. C., Bowman, M. B., & Harbin, H. T. (2019). Reimbursement of apps for mental health: Current practices and potential pathways. *JMIR Mental Health, 6*, e14724. https://doi.org/10.2196/14724

Public Health Emergency. (n.d.). *Waiver or Modification of Requirements Under Section 1135 of the Social Security Act.* https://www.phe.gov/emergency/news/healthactions/section1135/Pages/covid19-13March20.aspx

Shah, S. J., Schwamm, L. H., Cohen, A. B., Simoni, M. R., Estrada, J., Matiello, M., & Rao, S. K. (2018). Virtual visits partially replaced in-person visits in an ACO-based medical specialty practice. *Health Affairs, 37*(12), 2045–2051. https://doi.org/10.1377/hlthaff.2018.05105

United Nations. (2020, May 13). *Policy brief: COVID-19 and the need for action on mental health.* https://www.un.org/sites/un2.un.org/files/un_policy_brief-covid_and_mental_health_final.pdf

US Food and Drug Administration. (n.d.). *BeSafeRx: Know your online pharmacy.* https://www.fda.gov/drugs/besaferx-know-your-online-pharmacy/media#7

World Health Organization. (2020, May 14). *News release.* https://www.who.int/news-room/detail/14-05-2020-substantial-investment-needed-to-avert-mental-health-crisis

FINANCIAL MANAGEMENT

LEARNING OBJECTIVES

1. Explain the key components of **revenue cycle** management in ambulatory care
2. Understand how to effectively manage expenses in the ambulatory care setting with consideration to fixed and variable costs
3. Recognize the various types of financial statements and their use cases

KEY TERMS

Revenue Cycle	Provider-Based Clinic
Payer	Denial
Gross Charge	Fixed Costs
Allowable	Profit
Eligibility	Overhead
Financial Clearance	

INTRODUCTION

Financial management of the ambulatory practice includes the standard financial and accounting functions required of a business enterprise, as well as the management of a complex revenue cycle that involves billing for healthcare services and ensuring timely and appropriate remuneration from government **payers**, insurance payers, and patients.

REVENUE

Optimizing the revenue of an ambulatory practice is arguably the most crucial responsibility of leadership. This task is particularly challenging as revenue is one of the most complex and contentious management issues in a practice as a result of the highly regulated environment in which practices operate. Most ambulatory practices are paid based on the delivery of a service or product to a patient. For example, an orthopaedic practice bills and collects for an encounter that features the evaluation and management of a patient presenting with a sprained wrist, to include an X-ray and a brace. If the service is scheduled but never rendered, it is not paid. That is, a patient who is scheduled for a visit but does not arrive for the visit results in zero revenue to an ambulatory practice. The term *fee for service* (FFS) emanates from this concept as monies are received only upon the provision of services. In an FFS environment, the *volume of services* produced is crucial to revenue.

Reimbursement Models

Increasingly, alternative reimbursement methodologies are replacing the historically dominant paradigm of FFS revenue, although a link to services performed on behalf of patients for which the ambulatory practice cares remains in all reimbursement models. Alternative payment schemes are proliferating as the healthcare industry focuses on delivering value and controlling costs; examples include the following:

Flat monthly payment: There may be a level monthly payment for patients who are assigned to the practice; this is common in primary care and is often called a "per member per month" payment. The payment may vary based on the patient's acuity or other factors as dictated by the payer.

Episodes of care: The practice may be paid a set amount based on an entire episode of care related to a particular diagnosis, disease, or surgical intervention. As an example, a total hip replacement procedure may be reimbursed at a set fee, regardless of each of the Current Procedural Terminology (CPT) codes captured in the preoperative, operative, and postoperative periods. This model of reimbursement is standard for the physician's professional services as it relates to surgeries and many procedures. The mechanism is referred to as a global fee or payment, since it encompasses the service in its entirety, from beginning to end. Surgeries and procedures are designated as minor or major, with the duration of 10 or 90 days, respectively. All services within that period are included in the global payment, with limited exceptions. This model has been common industry practice for payers' reimbursement of the services of surgeons but is expanding to encompass associated services. For example, the payer may allocate a single fee for the total hip replacement that incorporates the surgeon, as well as the hospital, an anesthesiologist, a pathologist, a radiologist, rehabilitation, therapy—and any other service that is involved in the patient's treatment. Reimbursement for CPT–International Statistical Classification of Diseases and Related Health Problems (ICD) code linkages may override the contracted **allowable** rates for individual CPT codes, thereby reimbursing the amount the payer deems appropriate for the management of the patient's condition.

Risk payments and takebacks: There may also be additional payments—or takebacks of money—if the practice bears financial risk for the patient's care. Extra payments are made if the care is managed within a given threshold—or the monies may be extracted or withheld if risk-based targets are not met.

Bonus payments: Other arrangements may include bonus payments for meeting quality or patient experience metrics or for meeting targets and goals associated with reimbursement levels. These, too, are typically established and managed by the payer. Varying in construct, the bonus payments may be offered at the physician or provider level but are more typically a function of the entire practice's performance. If the latter, there may be an exertion of peer pressure to address the parameters of the reimbursement model.

There is no standard approach to a reimbursement model; ambulatory practices may face a variety of payment relationships. Recording revenue may require consultation with an accountant, as well as consideration of the manner in which the monies can be best incorporated in management reporting. Furthermore, at a tactical level, there may be considerations regarding the reconciliation of revenue to the expected services.

Net Patient Services Revenue

There may be additional sources of nonpatient care revenue, such as grants, contracts, directorship fees, or expert witness fees; however, most revenue is associated with billing and collections for professional services (those generated by clinicians as they provide patient care) and for technical services (those generated through facilities or equipment that allow for separate reimbursement). Together, the professional and technical revenue is referred to as "net patient services revenue" (NPSR). In the case of the patient with the sprained wrist, the ambulatory practice received revenue for the surgeon's evaluation and management and the imaging study, as well as the brace that was provided to the patient.

A dollar for a service is a dollar for a service, correct? Not in an ambulatory practice. Payment for healthcare services is vastly different from consumer markets. When a customer enters a store to purchase a loaf of bread, the customer expects to pay the price posted for the bread. In contrast, the nature of the demand for healthcare services is random; illness, injury, and life-threatening emergencies are often unpredictable. Emergency hospitalizations, surgery, rehabilitation services, and other advanced treatments can be very costly to pay for out of pocket. As a result, patients obtain health insurance as a means of mitigating personal financial risk. Being insured is of such import that employers offer it as a benefit to attract and retain employees. The main premise of health insurance is that it allows for the risk pooling of groups of individuals; a similar analogy is observed with other insurance offerings, such as automobile insurance. Although insurance is an individual decision, many patients maintain insurance coverage for healthcare services. Therefore, health insurance is an essential component of revenue for an ambulatory practice. Because health insurance companies are buying services from practices, an insurance company is often referred to as a "payer" by the ambulatory practice.

Payer Mix

The mixture of health insurance companies, including the government, commercial companies, and patients who are financially responsible for their own care, is a factor impacting the revenue performance of an ambulatory practice. Collectively, the ambulatory practice's book of business is referred to as the practice's *payer mix*. Figure 6.1 displays a sample payer mix, noting that there is no standard, industry-wide categorization of insurance companies. Some practices report Medicare, Medicaid, Workers' Compensation, Tricare, and other government payers as "Government" while others break down each of these payers—and those in the commercial sector—into a separate category. Payer mix is formulated and displayed based on **gross charges** due to the normalization of data; that is, a 99213 is always $150 for the practice (if that represents its charge for 99213), regardless of the reimbursement that is based on the patient's coverage and practice-payer contracted rate (The reimbursement is represented by the allowable, a concept discussed in detail later).

The ambulatory practice's payer mix influences revenue because of the variance in reimbursement. Some payers contribute a higher payment amount to the practice per unit of service. In this case, a shift of business to that particular insurer may result in higher total revenue. Importantly, this dynamic may occur without any additional cost to the practice. For example, let's assume that the allowable for the American

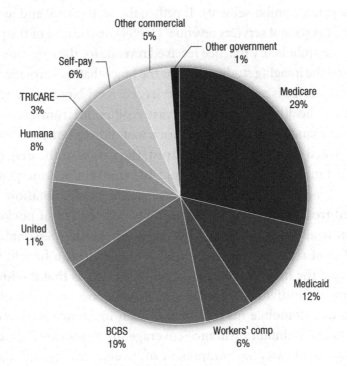

FIGURE 6.1 Payer mix distribution (sample).

BCBS, Blue Cross Blue Shield; comp, compensation.

Insurance Preferred Provider Organization (PPO) plan is $84.50 for a 99213, but it is $124.50 for Regional Platinum. The service costs the same to produce for a patient covered by American Insurance as that for a patient covered by Regional Platinum. If two Regional Platinum patients were seen instead of the current combination of one patient from each payer, an additional $40 of revenue could be collected due to the change in payer mix. Alternatively, the practice may calculate that 10% of its patient base is covered by Umbrella Insurance. As this represents the single largest insurer for the practice, efforts may be made by the practice to communicate with Umbrella to renegotiate the allowables to more favorable reimbursement levels.

The management of payer mix is challenging for ambulatory practices as the mixture of payers is often a reflection of the community surrounding the practice rather than efforts made by the practice. For example, a practice situated in a geographic area that is mainly retirees will likely maintain a payer mix that is dominated by the federal insurance for persons aged 65 and older in the United States, Medicare. Payer mix is not impossible to affect, however. The practice may market its services to a targeted patient base, initiate a branding strategy in an adjacent community, or open a satellite location to attract patients who may be covered by a payer with more favorable reimbursement.

Gross Charge

Ambulatory practices maintain a fee schedule that outlines the prices for each unit of service. These prices are referred to as "gross charges" in ambulatory practices; most ambulatory practices have a standard fee schedule that outlines the "gross charge"— which may also be referred to as the "charge" or "fee"—for each unit of service it offers. These may be maintained privately (releasing only the services that the patient receives) or posted for public viewing. Increasingly, patients are demanding transparency of pricing; such expectations may be supported by legal requirements for transparency at the federal or state level.

Unlike most other goods and services, remuneration for the specific unit of service in an ambulatory practice is rarely equal to its stated gross charge. Instead, revenue received for the service varies based on contracts that the practice has entered into with insurance companies, often denoted as "payers." There may be a single contract or hundreds. Reimbursement rates, referred to as "allowable rates" or "allowables," differ by payer and within a particular payer by health plan and/or employer contract.

Further complicating the determination of the accurate reimbursement for a particular service, many of the payers have rules related to the elements of a service, for example, the services that are to be bundled with a particular CPT code, such as a test with an encounter, and other payment modifications based on the volume, frequency, and nature of services rendered. Additionally, the ambulatory practice may not receive an explicit reimbursement schedule from the payer that links reimbursement to each unit of service; instead, the contract may be based on a percentage of another payer's allowables, such as a percentage of Medicare allowables. Furthermore, payers may maintain rules related to levels of copayment, deductibles, and coinsurance that must be collected from the insurance company's beneficiary—the patient—often before the insurance company paying

EXHIBIT 6.1 PATIENT FINANCIAL RESPONSIBILITY: COMMON TERMS

Copayment: A set fee or a percentage of the allowable that is to be collected by the practice for the patient's visit, often established based on visit type. As an example, a patient may be required to pay a $50 copayment each time he or she has a face-to-face visit with the physician.

Deductible: A financial threshold expected to be paid by the patient prior to insurance paying for healthcare services. As an example, the patient may have a policy with a $2,500 deductible. Until the deductible has been "met" (translated as paid by the patient), the insurance company is not responsible for payment. Many health plans have multiple deductible tiers—for example, there can be tiers based on in-network and out-of-network services, as well as at the individual and family level.

Coinsurance: The percentage of payment the patient is expected to pay for a particular service. In essence, the patient's insurance company has determined that it and the patient will "co-insure" or pay together for a particular service. Coinsurance is often 20% of the allowable; it is typically imposed after the deductible is met.

Out of Network: The health plan offers levels of coverage in conjunction with the provider and facility network offered by the insurance company. If the patient chooses to receive a service outside of the insurance company's designated network, the patient may have a higher level of cost sharing.

Out-of-Pocket Maximum: An established amount in a given year, which may be tiered based on a family unit and each individual within it, that provides a cumulative threshold under which the patient owes payment. Once the maximum is met based on a combination of the deductible, coinsurance, and copayment amounts, the insurance company pays the remaining balance.

Noncovered Services: The health plan provides coverage for a select set of services; if the patient receives a service that is outside of the parameters of the select services, the patient may be financially responsible for the services. This may include, but not be limited to, services that are not considered medically necessary by the payer such as an experimental procedure, administrative fees such as paperwork completion, specific services that are not included in the plan such as fertility treatments, or limits on the number visits that a patient can have for selected services.

its share of the allowable. Exhibit 6.1 defines these out-of-pocket patient payments often required of patients according to the construct of their health plan; collectively, these represent the patient's cost share. These reimbursement nuances do not represent an exhaustive list; ambulatory practices face an ever-evolving payment environment.

Determining whether the ambulatory practice has optimized its reimbursement from all potential payment sources—the patient, the government, and commercial payers—is complex. A successful outcome requires that the patient and the practice be informed regarding the patient's insurance and the patient's out-of-pocket payment obligations—and take appropriate action to successfully collect the expected financial obligations from all parties. Optimal reimbursement practices are achieved by understanding and complying with a complex web of reimbursement issues inherent to ambulatory practices—and executing them successfully.

REVENUE CYCLE

An overview of the typical process of billing for a rendered service and collecting reimbursement for a healthcare service in an ambulatory practice is reported in Figure 6.2. The entire process is referred to as the practice's "revenue cycle;" consequently, the handling of the process is known as "revenue cycle management" (RCM). Some of the revenue cycle functions are conducted at the practice site, such as verifying the patient's insurance and plan (referred to as the "**eligibility** process"), collecting patient out-of-pocket payments, and capturing and coding charges. Others are performed by personnel in the practice's business office or billing service, such as claim submission, claim follow-up, payment posting, and reimbursement analysis.

The following sections describe the key components of the revenue cycle process involved in translating a service into final payment.

Pre-Visit

The initial stage of the revenue cycle occurs prior to rendering a service. Often referred to as the **financial clearance** process, the pre-visit step establishes the framework for a successful outcome to the revenue cycle. Not only does an effective pre-visit process facilitate accurate and timely payment for the practice, but it also enables the practice to service the patient's financial health successfully. If the practice misses an element of the patient's insurance, the billing process breaks down—and the patient receives a bill for the full charge. In addition to the registration process, which collectively involves capturing and confirming the demographic and insurance information for the patient, the pre-visit process incorporates engaging with the patient about their financial responsibility—and collecting, as appropriate.

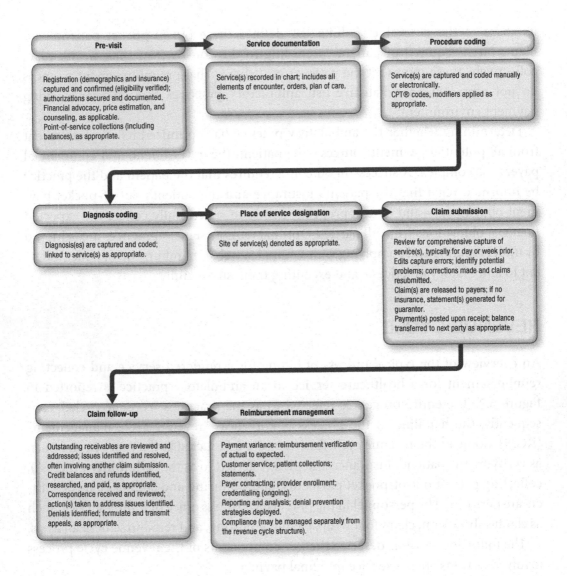

FIGURE 6.2 Ambulatory practice revenue cycle.

Service Documentation

To permit billing and collection of the clinical service, the service must be documented. The note is most often recorded in the patient's electronic health record. Enhancing the accuracy and specificity of encounter documentation is a heightened focus for ambulatory practices. Termed *clinical documentation improvement* (CDI), these efforts target clinicians for training and education to permit the creation of an accurate patient record that reflects all aspects of the care provided. There are many benefits related to CDI, including ensuring high-quality care in the patient's healthcare journey. From a business perspective, one of the many advantages is the creation of a document that supports accurate coding. Correct coding facilitates timely and accurate reimbursement, as well as provides documentation support in the event the payer denies payment for services and the practice needs to appeal the denied claim.

Procedure Coding

Procedure coding involves assigning a specific procedure code to each service that was performed and documented. A procedure code must be affixed to the service to permit billing and reimbursement to occur.

Historically, clinicians would simply record the services they performed—for example, "I treated the patient for a cold." But what exactly does that mean? One physician may have spent minutes with the patient, looking them up and down and telling them to go home and have some soup. Another clinician may have spent hours examining and assessing the patient, determining and addressing the social determinants of health that may affect the patient, ordering tests, creating a plan, counseling the patient, and coordinating the patient's care. The reality is that "I treated the patient for a cold" likely falls somewhere between these scenarios, but it demonstrates the difficulty of translating a clinician's notes into payment.

To create structure and consistency within the reimbursement system, the American Medical Association (AMA) formulated procedure codes by introducing the CPT code set in 1966. Originally only incorporating surgical procedures, the code set was broadened in the subsequent decades to incorporate all professional medical services. The predecessor of the Centers for Medicare and Medicaid Services (CMS) adopted CPT as a component of the federal agency's Healthcare Common Procedure Coding System (HCPCS).

CPT presides today as one of the principal code sets. The code set was promulgated to this status as it was the centerpiece of the federal government's mandate to establish electronic transaction standards per the Health Insurance Portability and Accountability Act (HIPAA) of 1996. CPT officially became the national coding standard for professional medical services and procedures in 2000; the code set continues to be maintained by the AMA and updated on an annual basis. CPT codes feature a total of five digits. The main set, Category I codes, is numeric, while supplemental Category II and III codes are a combination of numeric and alphabetic characters. The CPT code may be altered by one of dozens of modifiers. The two-digit modifier, which follows the CPT code and is typically separated by a hyphen, may change the payment or be used for informational purposes only. It is important to note that there is only one CPT code set used by all clinicians; in other words, CPT is specialty-agnostic. Therefore, the same CPT code may be used by an internist or a neurologist, for example, and it must represent the same service as per the description of the code.

In the previously discussed scenario about a patient being treated for a cold, the clinician would likely use a code from the evaluation and management (E&M) section of CPT codebook. The clinician would necessarily review their documented actions to determine which code to select. As an example, CPT code 99213, one of the most frequently used codes, represents an office or other outpatient visit for evaluation and management of an established patient. Box 6.1 features the description of this CPT code.

Diagnosis Coding

Now that the service has been documented and a CPT code assigned, the unit of service must then be matched—referred to as "linked"—with a diagnosis code that signals the patient's diagnosis or reason for service. The diagnosis coding system that is employed is the ICD. This medical classification list is authored and maintained by the World Health Organization (WHO). In 2015, the United States adopted the 10th revision of its national ICD variant, the Clinical Modification version. This diagnosis coding set, which contains approximately 70,000 codes, is referred to as International Classification of Diseases, Tenth Revision, Clinical Modification (ICD-10-CM).

Each procedure CPT code is linked to one or more ICD-10-CM codes. The ICD-10-CM code may represent the diagnosis for the treatment related to the encounter; however, it may also represent supplemental, but important, information about the patient. ICD-10-CM codes can represent etiology and manifestations, sequelae, external causes of morbidity and mortality, and factors influencing the patient's health status. The ICD, according to the WHO (n.d.), is the "foundation for the identification of health trends and statistics globally, and the international standard for reporting diseases and health conditions." The codes are also used for clinical and research purposes to further improvements to public health.

In contrast to the varying code sets to describe services (e.g., the diagnosis-related groups [DRGs] is used by hospitals, while CPT is the code set for clinicians rendering

---

| BOX 6.1 | DESCRIPTION OF CPT 99213 |

Office or other outpatient visit for the evaluation and management of an established patient, which requires a medical appropriate history and/or examination and low level of medical decision making. When using time for code selection, 20–29 minutes of total time is spent on the date of the encounter.

SOURCE: American Medical Association. (2021). *CPT® 2021*.

professional services), all healthcare entities that provide services in the United States use ICD-10-CM to express the diagnosis (or diagnoses) for payment purposes.

Although the discussion of coding herein refers to procedure coding preceding diagnosis coding, the order may be reversed—or both codes may be selected simultaneously.

Resource-Based Relative Value Scale

The resource-based relative value scale (RBRVS) was created in the late 1980s as an objective payment mechanism for Medicare reimbursement for professional services, a key offering of ambulatory practices. Until the launch of the scale in 1992 for reimbursement, Medicare was paying a percentage of the practice's charge for the unit of service. If the practice charged $100 for a CPT, Medicare would pay some portion of that—let's assume 80%—and the allowable would therefore be $80. Although ubiquitous for many years, this method proved to be unsustainable as clinicians could simply raise their charges to garner additional payment.

The RBRVS features a unit—a total relative value unit (RVU)—associated with each CPT code. The total RVU is constructed from three components: work effort, practice expense, and malpractice. Each component is adjusted based on geography. The sum of the components—the total RVU—is multiplied by a payment conversion factor that is updated annually by the federal government. The calculation results in the Medicare allowable for each CPT code. See Figure 6.3: Payment Formula using RBRVS.

Soon after the launch of the scale, Medicare was joined by other insurance companies embracing the RBRVS as a basis for professional services reimbursement. Today, the RBRVS provides the foundation for the majority of insurance payments for professional services. The RBRVS is not without its challenges, however.[1]

The work RVU, one of the three components of the total RVU, is commonly used for capturing, monitoring, and analyzing clinician productivity. It also serves as a basis for cost accounting, cost allocation, and many other analyses as it accounts for the work associated with the unit of service without regard to the payment. This means that a service can be counted equally whether it is performed for an American Insurance or Regional Platinum patient – or a patient who does not pay at all. In sum, it liberates the service from its payment, making it useful for a wide range of analyses.

---

[1] Challenges associated with the RBRVS include, but are not limited to, the fact that the scale is updated each year, creating issues for trend analyses; there are not units associated with every CPT® code, particularly those not considered payable by Medicare; and there are stakeholders who disagree with the assigned values associated with the codes, especially the work component. Despite these challenges, the scale is the industry standard and allows internal and external comparisons.

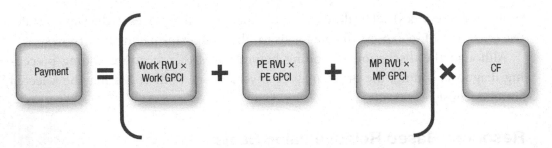

FIGURE 6.3 Payment formula for the resource-based relative value scale (RBRVS).

RVU, relative value unit; CF, conversion factor; GPCI, geographic practice cost index; MP, malpractice; PE, practice expense
SOURCE: Centers for Medicare and Medicaid Services. (n.d.). *How to use the searchable Medicare Physician Fee Schedule.* https://www.cms.gov/files/document/2020-physician-fee-schedule-guide.pdf

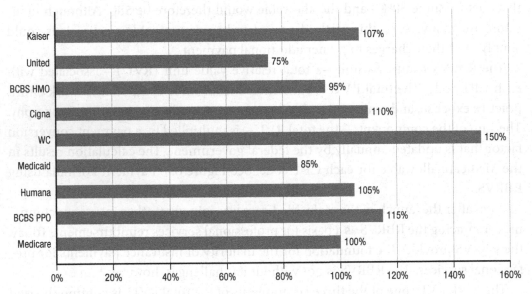

FIGURE 6.4 Sample analysis: reimbursement by payer as compared to Medicare.

BCBS, Blue Cross Blue Shield; HMO, Health Maintenance Organization; PPO: Preferred Provider Organization; WC, Workers' Compensation

The complexity of the reimbursement system makes the payer mix, and the impact of a shift, difficult to evaluate. Therefore, the practice may utilize the RBRVS for further analysis. A sample analysis is displayed in Figure 6.4; Medicare's RBRVS is used as the baseline, allowing for direct comparison across payers.

Place of Service Designation

Ambulatory practices may operate in a variety of practice sites and facilities. These facilities are referred to using "place of service" (POS) codes. Reimbursement differs based on the site on which the services were performed. Thus, the POS must also be coded for the unit of service and submitted in the appropriate field on the billing claim form to permit appropriate billing and reimbursement.

A list of the common POS codes identifying settings in which ambulatory practices operate is provided in Exhibit 6.2.

EXHIBIT 6.2 PARTIAL LISTING OF PLACE OF SERVICE CODES AND DESCRIPTIONS FOR PROFESSIONAL CLAIMS IN AMBULATORY SETTINGS

11 Office Location. Office location other than a hospital, skilled nursing facility (SNF), military treatment facility, community health center, state or local public health clinic, or intermediate care facility (ICF), where the health professional routinely provides health examinations, diagnosis, and treatment of illness or injury on an ambulatory basis.

12 Home Location. Home location other than a hospital or other facility, where the patient receives care in a private residence.

15 Mobile Unit. A facility/unit that moves from place to place equipped to provide preventive, screening, diagnostic, and/or treatment services.

17 Walk-In Retail Health Clinic. A walk-in health clinic, other than an office, urgent care facility, pharmacy, or independent clinic and not described by any other POS code that is located within a retail operation and provides, on an ambulatory basis, preventive and primary care services.

19 Off-Campus Outpatient Hospital. A portion of an off-campus hospital provider-based department that provides diagnostic, therapeutic (both surgical and nonsurgical), and rehabilitation services to sick or injured persons who do not require hospitalization or institutionalization.

20 Urgent Care Facility Location. Distinct from a hospital emergency room, an office, or a clinic, whose purpose is to diagnose and treat illness or injury for unscheduled, ambulatory patients seeking immediate medical attention.

22 On-Campus Outpatient Hospital. A portion of a hospital's main campus that provides diagnostic, therapeutic (both surgical and nonsurgical), and rehabilitation services to sick or injured persons who do not require hospitalization or institutionalization.

24 Ambulatory Surgical Center. A freestanding facility, other than a physician's office, where surgical and diagnostic services are provided on an ambulatory basis.

50 Federally Qualified Health Center. A facility located in a medically underserved area that provides Medicare beneficiaries preventive primary medical care under the general direction of a physician.

SOURCE: Centers for Medicare and Medicaid Services. (2019, October). Place of service codes for professional claims database. https://www.cms.gov/Medicare/Coding/place-of-service-codes/Place_of_Service_Code_Set

For this chapter, the details of reimbursement related to the four ambulatory places of service with the highest volume—doctors' offices (11); hospital outpatient clinics (19 and 22); and ambulatory surgery centers (24)—are described in detail.

Place of service 11 describes clinicians' offices, regardless of ownership. These ambulatory practices use a CPT for billing purposes, with billing submitted on a CMS-1500 claim form. The Medicare Physician Fee Schedule (PFS) is used for reimbursement. Collectively, the services that are rendered are considered "professional services." In addition to physicians, other healthcare professionals bill and collect services using this POS.

Places of service 19 and 22 reflect hospital outpatient clinics; ownership of the practice is a critical factor with a hospital or health system serving as the owner. A hospital outpatient clinic must be credentialed as a hospital outpatient clinic with Medicare, Medicaid, and other payers and follow rules and regulations issued for this designation (e.g., compliance with the Joint Commission), except in extenuating circumstances. If recognized as a hospital outpatient clinic, the practice uses a CPT code to indicate the professional service on a CMS-1500 form, and it also bills a facility charge which is documented and submitted on a different claim form—the CMS-1450 (UB-04). The professional services are paid at a lower rate than a professional service rendered in a non-facility setting like a doctor's office (11). In addition to professional services, the hospital outpatient clinic is paid a flat fee for the use of the facility in which that service is performed. POS 19 indicates the clinic is off-campus; POS 22 signals an on-campus clinic. The facility charge may or may not be paid by insurance companies other than Medicare and Medicaid. This form of practice configuration is referred to by several names, most commonly, "**provider-based clinic**" or "hospital-based clinic." Furthermore, the term *split billing* may be referenced because two claims—the professional fee and the facility charge—are submitted.

Place of service 24 indicates services performed in an ambulatory surgery center (ASC). Like the hospital outpatient clinics, the entity must be credentialed and recognized as an ASC. Although the professional services are billed using CPT codes, the facility fee differs. ASCs are paid using a distinct reimbursement mechanism called the Outpatient Prospective Payment System (OPPS). More information about the OPPS can be found in Exhibit 6.3.

For the ambulatory practices that incorporate professional and facility services, there may be two distinct entities involved in the revenue cycle. For example, an academic faculty practice plan may house its oncology practice in a hospital outpatient clinic; the practice plan would then bill the professional service, while the university hospital billed the facility fee. The same scenario may hold true with an ASC. Alternatively, if a single entity has ownership of the clinicians and the facility, the billing may be performed by the same entity. Therefore, the correct place of service is considered a crucial factor for ambulatory practices, particularly due to its influence on revenue.

EXHIBIT 6.3 OUTPATIENT PROSPECTIVE PAYMENT SYSTEM

The Outpatient Prospective Payment System (OPPS) provides the payment structure for the facility fee associated with hospital outpatient services. Commenced in 2000, OPPS replaced a payment system that was formulated based on hospital-reported costs. Like professional services, OPPS establishes payment according to a conversion factor and relative weights, with an adjustment for geography. The conversion factor, which is updated annually by the hospital market basket index less a multifactor productivity adjustment, is affected by the hospitals' successful reporting on quality metrics.

Unlike the PFS, hospitals may be eligible for outlier payment adjustments for high-cost services, as well as pass-through reimbursement for novel technology. At the passage of OPPS, there were some exceptions made for select cancer, rural, and children's hospitals with a positive payment modifier, and these concessions remain. Figure 6.5 illustrates the OPPS.

The CMS categorizes individual services into ambulatory payment classifications (APCs) based on clinical characteristics and cost similarity. The services within an APC have the same rate; APCs are reviewed and updated by an expert provider advisory panel. New technology APCs are established each year, with the services remaining in the classification for two to three years to allow CMS adequate time to research and value the services for payment. Separate payment is made for blood, blood products, and some drugs, among others. The APC does not include professional services. Ancillary services—those that are supportive or adjunctive—to a procedure are incorporated into the payment for the primary service; this form of packaging is to encourage hospitals to effectively use resources. For the clinic encounter, off-campus, provider-based hospital outpatient clinics are paid based on a PFS-equivalent payment rate. Hospital clinics on or near—250 yards—campus remain on the OPPS program. These rules are subject to change.

Claim Submission

The CPT code, its corresponding diagnosis(es), and place of service are then submitted for reimbursement on the appropriate claim form. Typically, the information is transmitted through the practice's information system.[2] Accompanied by several

---

[2] This step often involves several processes, including manual intervention; for some ambulatory practices, the clinician may be alerted of the possible codes associated with the services rendered on the basis of the clinician's documentation; for other practices, a designated coding expert—a "coder"—may fully abstract the record and select the appropriate codes. Some ambulatory practices use a combination of these approaches or choose an intervention that features an audit of a portion of the encounters. After the codes are selected, they are entered or approved and then released for billing. While most practices have a combined information system, some practices may have a practice management system, in addition to an electronic health record system. Thus, the term *system* used herein is not meant to describe a specific product or solution but rather may involve several manual and/or electronic steps.

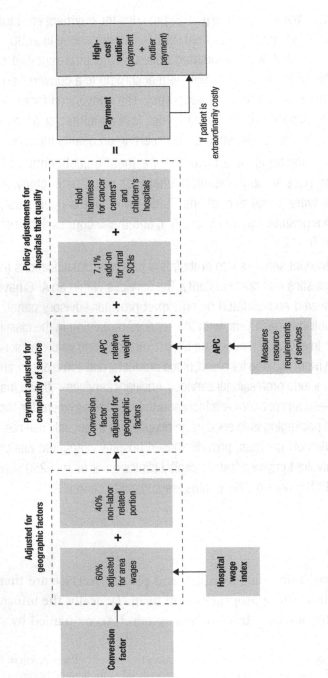

FIGURE 6.5 The outpatient prospective payment system.

SOURCE: Medicare Payment Advisory Commission. (2016, October). *Outpatient hospital services payment system* (p. 2). http://www.medpac.gov/docs/default-source/payment-basics/medpac_payment_basics_16_opd_final.pdf

NOTE: The ambulatory payment classification is the service classification system for the outpatient prospective payment system.
*Medicare adjusts outpatient prospective payment system payment rates for 11 cancer centers so that the payment-to-cost ratio (PCR) for each cancer center is equal to the average PCR for all hospitals.
APC, ambulatory payment classification; SCH, sole community hospital.

dozen other data elements—such as the patient's name, date of birth, the date the service was rendered, and so forth—the claim is transmitted to an insurance company for adjudication. The transmission is most often electronic, traveling from the practice's system through a clearinghouse via electronic data interchange (EDI) to reach the correct party for payment. In sending the information to the payer, the clearinghouse may halt the data from transmitting should errors be identified, instead deliver an electronic report back to the ambulatory practice for billing personnel to review and resolve. This document—often referred to as the edit or error report—is essential for the practice personnel to work so that the claims may be subsequently released and successfully transmitted to the appropriate payers.

If no insurance is involved, that is, the patient is "self-pay," the information about the service is placed on a statement that is transmitted to the guarantor—the person responsible for the patient's financial obligation. This financially responsible party is often the patient but may also be the patient's spouse or parent. A claim is an invoice seeking payment from the payer; a statement is an invoice seeking payment from the patient.

Claim Follow-Up

After the claim is submitted, the ambulatory practice must follow up with the government and private payers to ensure that the claim is paid; many of the private payers have timely filing claim requirements that must be met if the practice is to be paid. Although the deadlines are issued by the payer and thus vary, they are typically 60 to 90 days, with 365 days being a threshold for many government payers. Ambulatory practice personnel must also follow up with guarantors or patients to ensure statements are paid. An ambulatory practice actively manages outstanding insurance collections and patient collections, collectively known as its *accounts receivables*. The accounts receivables are typically reported by the payer, and aggregated by payer type, to permit effective analysis of outstanding payment levels. An associated report, the aged trial balance (ATB), provides the practice with knowledge related to the aging of the outstanding receivables. A sample ATB is presented in Table 6.1. In addition to the ATB, a report that calculates the days in receivables outstanding (DRO) serves as a key performance indicator (KPI). The DRO is calculated by dividing the total current receivables (net of credits) by the current average daily charge; additional information about KPIs is highlighted later.

Personnel in the practice's business office (or via a vendor billing service) conduct systematic work processes to identify and manage aged accounts receivables. (See the sidebar "From the Experts" for recommendations of best practices by ambulatory practice billing experts.) Payments may be delayed for a variety of reasons to include ineffective claim transmission, pending claim edits, claim **denials**, payer requests for additional information, and a host of other reasons. Because the guarantor (patient

TABLE 6.1 Sample Aged Trial Balance

DAYS OUTSTANDING	RECEIVABLES	PERCENTAGE
0–30	$19,110,769	75.53
31–60	$2,197,524	8.69
61–90	$1,153,465	4.56
91–120	$705,772	2.79
121–150	$507,969	2.01
151–180	$366,722	1.45
181+	$1,260,015	4.98
TOTAL	$25,302,236	100.00

or patient's responsible party) is typically also paying for the service (a copayment, deductible, coinsurance, or balance), the ability to collect from the patient is also critical to achieving the full payment. Reimbursement levels, particularly patient receivables, naturally decline with the aging of the accounts receivables. This stage may also address credit balances and refunds—monies that are due to be returned to the appropriate party, a common occurrence given the complexity of the revenue cycle.

Collecting these outstanding amounts from payers and patients is the responsibility of the ambulatory practice's business office[3] or vendor, often referred to as a billing service.

FROM THE EXPERTS: REVENUE CYCLE MANAGEMENT BEST PRACTICES

Mona Reimers, MBA

Director of Administrative Operations

Mary Ellen Kellogg

Billing Office Supervisor

Ortho NorthEast

Fort Wayne, Indiana

Managing the revenue cycle of an ambulatory practice isn't easy, but there are some themes that facilitate better outcomes. Here's our top 10 list of RCM best practices.

---

[3] There are several terms for this group of personnel in an ambulatory practice: In addition to the business office, the name of the collective team may be billing office or department or revenue cycle office or department. The duties may incorporate all aspects of the revenue cycle or just components of it. If tasks are allocated, it is often the tasks associated with addressing claims after they have been prepared and submitted.

1. *Maintain proof.* Billing can get messy; follow-up is often required. Electronic data interchange transactions are standardized data exchanges with time- and date-stamped receipts that can help a practice prove its claims are filed on time.

2. *Report metrics.* Strong financials rely on tracking key performance indicators from initial data entry about the patient to the point of care and to billing and follow-up. Dashboards provide practices with a high-level review to monitor progress and identify trends in numerous RCM variables, including staff production, collections, aging receivables, clean claim rates, charges, relative value units (RVUs), and so on.

3. *Know the rules.* Practices can avoid costly delays by becoming familiar with each payer's unique requirements for submitting clean claims. For example, some payers accept bilateral codes billed on one line with a −50 modifier while others want those codes listed as separate line items.

4. *Watch for underpayments.* After a payer has adjudicated the claim, the practice should verify that the claim was accurately processed and paid per contracted rates.

5. *Determine root cause.* Identifying the source of the error—a poor workflow or a onetime issue, for example—can help avoid future denials.

6. *Billing codes matter.* Payers use billing codes—CPT, ICD10, HCC, and so on—to assess the health of a practice's patient population and rate the quality of its providers. Even information from outside sources, such as a patient's hospital readmission after surgery, can factor into how the payer determines your providers' quality of care and, ultimately, their reimbursement.

7. *Manage denials.* By automatically checking each claim's accuracy before submission—suspending and returning those with missing or invalid information—practices can avoid denied claims, delayed payments, and the related costs of reworking inaccurate claims. Promptly reviewing claims that are denied or contain denied services is critical to filing timely appeals and avoiding underpayment or nonpayment for services.

8. *Recognize the interdependency.* Investing in the infrastructure of the workflow that generates the practice's revenue not only improves billing efficiency, but it also helps clinical and administrative staff make correct decisions as they contribute information into the workflow.

9. *Leverage technology.* Advances in technologies make it easier for patients to pay their portion in advance, online, by text, smartphone app, or by leaving credit card information on file with the practice.

10. *Engage the people.* Hiring positive personalities and measuring staff effectiveness and efficiency while providing consistent, ongoing staff training is vital to a practice's RCM success.

Reimbursement Management

The manner of routing the claim or statement to the responsible party is relatively simple, but the adjudication process introduces significant complexity. As discussed, the ambulatory practice has a gross charge for each unit of service and has contracted with payers to receive varying allowable rates for each service. The allowable represents the intended or expected payment. The allowable embodies what the term conveys—the allowable is what the practice can collect for the unit of service as defined by the CPT code, whether it is paid by the payer(s), the patient, or in combination. It is dictated by the contract into which practice has entered with the insurance company at the health plan level (with insurance companies offering a multitude of health plans). Therefore, a single insurance company may have multiple allowables for the same CPT code, with the patient's health plan determining the correct allowable to be paid.

The insurer may pay for some or all of this allowable, or it may indicate that the patient owes a portion (e.g., a copayment or coinsurance). Like the allowable, this may vary based on the plan—or even at the patient level—per the insurance policy purchased by the patient (or the patient's employer). Most payers will pay either the gross charge or the designated allowable, whichever is lower. Therefore, gross charges necessarily are monitored to exceed the highest intended payment from the insurance company.

Despite the best efforts an ambulatory practice may take to perform a service and to capture, code, and submit an accurate and timely claim, for an estimated 5% to 10% of service units, the insurance company denies payment altogether.[4] Common reasons and possible causes for denied claims are reported in Table 6.2. Identifying and analyzing denial reasons allows a practice to develop and execute plans to address the root causes of payment delays.

An ambulatory practice is presented with challenges related to payment; understanding and codifying denials allows a practice to address many of them. The denial may be valid—for example, the patient's insurance coverage expired, and this was not recognized by the practice—or it may represent a need for the practice to appeal for the service the practice considers it deserves to be paid. For example, the insurance company may deny payment for a service performed for a certain diagnosis, claiming that the service was not medically necessary. The practice may subsequently appeal the denied claim by elaborating on the nature of the patient's care that would permit the insurance company to reconsider and reverse its decision. Regardless of the particulars of a specific situation, denials offer a wealth of

---

[4] American Academy of Family Physicians. Revenue Cycle Management: Key Metrics. Accessed October 21, 2020, at https://www.aafp.org/family-physician/practice-and-career/managing-your-practice/practice -finances.html#

TABLE 6.2 Common Reasons and Possible Causes for Denied Claims

REASON FOR DENIAL	POSSIBLE CAUSES
PATIENT CANNOT BE IDENTIFIED AS OUR INSURED. CLAIM/SERVICE NOT COVERED BY THIS PAYER/CONTRACTOR YOU MUST SEND THE CLAIM/SERVICE TO THE CORRECT PAYER/CONTRACTOR. EXPENSES INCURRED AFTER COVERAGE TERMINATED. CLAIM SPANS INELIGIBLE AND ELIGIBLE PERIODS OF COVERAGE. REBILL SEPARATE CLAIMS. THIS CARE MAY BE COVERED BY ANOTHER PAYER PER COORDINATION OF BENEFITS.	The patients' insurance coverage was not collected or documented correctly; the patient reported having coverage that the patient did not have; insurance eligibility was not verified by the practice; the patient may have left the employer or switched insurance coverage or plans, but the payer's records do not reflect this change.
THE AUTHORIZATION NUMBER IS MISSING, INVALID, OR DOES NOT APPLY TO THE BILLED SERVICES OR PROVIDER. REFERRAL ABSENT OR EXCEEDED. SERVICES NOT AUTHORIZED BY NETWORK/ PRIMARY CARE PROVIDERS.	The practice failed to obtain the required authorization or referral for the services rendered or the valid referral period for the patient's health plan was exceeded.
THIS IS A NON-COVERED SERVICE BECAUSE IT IS A ROUTINE/PREVENTIVE EXAM OR A DIAGNOSTIC/SCREENING PROCEDURE DONE IN CONJUNCTION WITH A ROUTINE/ PREVENTIVE EXAM. THESE ARE NON-COVERED SERVICES BECAUSE THIS IS NOT DEEMED A "MEDICAL NECESSITY" BY THE PAYER. THE SERVICE/EQUIPMENT/DRUG IS NOT COVERED UNDER THE PATIENT'S CURRENT BENEFIT PLAN.	Not all services are covered by a patient's insurance policy. The practice did not verify coverage for services prior to being rendered to the patient. Patients with active health insurance have a variety of benefit structures as dictated by the health plan that they choose. If the patient was informed about the lack of or limited coverage or other arrangements were made, the financial responsibility for the service may be transferred to the patient or other guarantor.
CLAIM/SERVICE LACKS INFORMATION OR HAS SUBMISSION/BILLING ERROR(S), WHICH IS NEEDED FOR ADJUDICATION.	Data are missing from a field on the claim form, such as plan identification number, practice tax identification number, date of injury (for workers' compensation claim), rendering or referring physician's National Provider Identifier, and so forth. Pre-adjudication claim edits have not been established to the level of specificity required to ensure identification and correction of these errors prior to claim submission.

(continued)

TABLE 6.2 Common Reasons and Possible Causes for Denied Claims (*Continued*)

REASON FOR DENIAL	POSSIBLE CAUSES
PROCEDURE CODE WAS INVALID ON THE DATE OF SERVICE. THE PROCEDURE CODE IS INCONSISTENT WITH THE MODIFIER USED OR A REQUIRED MODIFIER IS MISSING. THE PROCEDURE CODE IS INCONSISTENT WITH THE PLACE OF SERVICE. THE PROCEDURE/REVENUE CODE IS INCONSISTENT WITH THE PATIENT'S AGE. THE DATE OF BIRTH FOLLOWS THE DATE OF SERVICE.	There are errors or omissions at coding, charge capture, or charge submission. Alternatively, there may be requirements of a payer related to the submission of data elements for payment of the service that are unknown or unmet.

SOURCE: Left column—data from Washington Publishing Company. (n.d.). *Claim adjustment reason codes.* https://x12.org/codes/claim-adjustment-reason-codes

information about payments and should be at the centerpiece of a practice's financial management strategy.

There are thousands of CPT and ICD-10-CM codes; most ambulatory practices handle hundreds of health plans. Scrutiny related to the correctness of payments is crucial to ensure that the intended payment is received; technology related to payment accuracy is all but necessary given the sheer volume of reimbursement possibilities. The expected "allowables" for each insurance company and health plan are typically loaded into the practice management system to crossmatch and verify that the amount paid is what is expected. Reimbursement levels that deviate from the expected allowables are then investigated by business office personnel to validate or appeal the payment levels.

Ambulatory practices may take the opportunity to negotiate higher payment rates. This may present in the format of seeking a boost to the allowables offered by an insurance company; alternatively, enhanced bundled payments, greater upside risk-sharing arrangements, or higher bonuses may be sought. Reimbursement may not always be the intended target of the negotiations; terms such as *timing of payment* or *reduction of administrative burden* may also be considerations. These negotiations may not always be successful; however, ambulatory practices that approach contract negotiations in a consistent, thoughtful manner are often rewarded with more favorable reimbursement.

A standard approach to measuring and monitoring practice management reports and key revenue cycle metrics aids in achieving optimal outcomes. Some of the key indicators include the following:

- Net collection rate (NCR): The net collection rate, one of the most often cited performance metrics for an ambulatory practice, is defined as NPSR divided by gross charges.

- Days in receivables outstanding (DRO): Total current accounts receivable (net of credits) divided by the average daily charge.

- ATB: Percentage of accounts receivable outstanding over a specified period of time (e.g., 90 to 120 days outstanding).

The revenue cycle is a critical function of a well-managed ambulatory practice. An effective approach to billing and collection requires attention to constructing and maintaining resources to permit timely and accurate attention to each step of the revenue cycle.

In summary, the revenue of an ambulatory practice results from a multitude of factors: volume, coding, place of service, reimbursement, collection/receivable management, and payer mix. The reimbursement landscape is ever-evolving, thereby creating a challenging, yet stimulating, environment.

EXPENSES

In an ambulatory practice, there is common treatment of the clinicians, support personnel, and management from an accounting perspective. The physicians are typically maintained as a separate line item; for a private practice, this is a result of their compensation being equal to the **profit** of the practice. In a practice in which the physicians are employed, the compensation may fluctuate based on productivity, quality, or other factors depending on their compensation model. Physicians, and sometimes advanced practice providers, are maintained separately from the support team, with the former category being documented distinctly as revenue generators, with the remaining personnel assisting those endeavors. Management may be incorporated in the support personnel category or identified as a separate line item.

Despite the differences in the composition and the size and type of support personnel, ambulatory practices typically spend a quarter of their revenue on the clinical and administrative workforce; this represents approximately half of the practice's investment in its **overhead**. Support personnel are often the single largest investment in resources to operate the practice.

Controlling costs is at the heart of running operations more smoothly and profitably in any type of business. Expenses—as defined by costs incurred to generate revenues—measure the resources, or assets, that an ambulatory practice uses to produce revenue. There are two broad categories of costs: fixed and variable.

Fixed Costs

Fixed costs—expenses that remain stable regardless of the ambulatory practice's volume—in an ambulatory practice may include the following:

- Personnel wages and benefits
- Technology (software and hardware)

- Furniture and equipment
- Building and occupancy (utilities, housekeeping, grounds, etc.)
- Professional liability and other insurance premiums
- Marketing
- Miscellaneous operating costs (e.g., administrative services) that do not depend on patient volume.

These fixed costs do not vary with the volume of patients. That is, if the volume of patients at a practice is 200 patients on Monday and 150 on Tuesday, the practice does not pay 25% less on Tuesday for its rent, telephones, personnel, liability insurance, and so on.

Step-Fixed Costs

A subdivision of fixed costs is step-fixed costs. These represent the costs that remain fixed until the volume of whatever activity they are supporting increases or decreases significantly; then the cost of that activity—the resources it uses—is adjusted up or down accordingly.

Personnel costs are considered step-fixed costs. Consider, for example, an ambulatory practice hires a new nurse practitioner. On the nurse practitioner's first day, the established team of personnel assigned to provide clinical support to the clinicians also assist the nurse practitioner. As the weeks go by, the nurse practitioner's schedule begins to fill. At some point in time, a new medical assistant is hired to support the nurse practitioner. Patient volume may trigger new personnel costs; other activities—portal messages, referrals, test results, and so forth—may also initiate the need to hire. Regardless of the activity that initiates the cost, the term *step* is used because the costs rise in a stepwise fashion, in contrast to a linear one.

Impact. There are two important points to remember about fixed and step-fixed costs:

Fixed and step-fixed costs do not change because of minor fluctuations in volume. That is, if the patient volume in an ambulatory practice increased from an average of 190 per day to 192 per day, the manager would not immediately hire another medical assistant.

Collectively, fixed and step-fixed costs account for most of the total operating cost structure in ambulatory practices. This creates a compelling opportunity for ambulatory practices to drive as much activity as possible through the operations of the practice, leveraging existing resources. For this strategy to be effective, the practice must strive to level-load the activity. For example, if a practice employs a team of five patient service representatives to receive and register patients as they arrive at the practice, the operation will be successful if the team processes 20 patients per hour at a steady pace throughout the day, instead of 40 in the first hour, five in the second,

50 in the third, and so forth. In this scenario, success is measured based on receiving and registering patients in a manner that is efficient and effective for the practice while minimizing the wait time for patients.

Variable Costs

Although most of the expenses of an ambulatory practice are fixed without regard to the volume of activity, other expenses occur only when a practice provides a service. These are the variable costs.

A variable cost is an expense that fluctuates based on the activity that caused the cost to occur in the first place. The activity, or resource consumption, that causes the majority of the variable costs in ambulatory practices is patient volume. To demonstrate what generally constitutes a variable cost, let us assume the service is a patient encounter. A disposable gown may be provided for the patient to wear for the encounter. The gown is an expense that occurred solely because of that patient encounter. This, and other activity-driven costs, are variable costs. Although most ambulatory practices have relatively few variable costs in comparison to fixed costs, the cost of medications and vaccines can be significant. Therefore, an oncology practice and a pediatric practice are careful not to expend a chemotherapy drug or an immunization, respectively, until the use of the resource is confirmed. Addressing workflow that leads to the spoilage of medications is an important consideration for an ambulatory practice aiming to control costs. Activity-based cost monitoring provides helpful insight regarding opportunities for financial improvement.

PROFIT

Revenue less expenses equals net income in an ambulatory practice. Although the definition is consistent, the net income, otherwise known as profit, may represent different outcomes. For an ambulatory practice that is owned and operated by an independent clinician, for example, profit equates to the money that he or she takes home as compensation. For some ambulatory practices, the clinician's compensation is embedded in the finances as a fixed cost. In this instance, any profit is used by the owner—a hospital, perhaps—to distribute as a bonus, fund an initiative, subsidize another part of the hospital, etc. Many ambulatory practices budget for breakeven—that is, the practice does not strive for a profit but rather focuses on generating sufficient revenue to cover the cost of the practice. The concept of overhead, furthermore, is important as the practice aims to effectively leverage its investment in infrastructure to facilitate optimal revenue. Like any business, the core concepts related to business profit apply to ambulatory practices; however, three topics—breakeven analysis, clinician compensation plans, and overhead— are of import for ambulatory practices.

Breakeven Analysis

Decision-making about costs in an ambulatory practice benefits from an understanding of calculating a breakeven volume point. The formula for breakeven volume:

$$(FC + PC) / (RE – VCE)^5 = Breakeven\ Volume,$$

where

>   FC = fixed costs,
>   PC = physician compensation,
>   RE = revenue per encounter, and
>   VCE = variable costs per encounter.

To illustrate the breakeven volume formula, let's assume the following:

>   Fixed costs = $20,000 per month
>   Physician compensation = $15,000 per month
>   Revenue per encounter = $150
>   Variable costs per encounter = $15

First, let us consider what variable we are solving for. We have the total costs for the practice (FC and PC), and we know what the practice is paid—and spends—per encounter, but how many encounters does the practice need to sustain this infrastructure? In other words, how many patients do we need to see to cover the practice's infrastructure (i.e., fixed costs) and physician compensation?

The element of time is vital. If the practice is estimating the breakeven volume for the year, the fixed costs and physician compensation in the scenario would first be multiplied by 12.

$$(\$35,000 \times 12)\ divided\ by\ (\$150–\$15) = 3,111$$

The breakeven volume is 3,111, meaning that the practice would need 3,111 encounters per year to cover the fixed costs of $20,000 per month and the physician compensation of $15,000 per month.

The next step involves translating this to a monthly, weekly, or daily data point. An ambulatory practice is typically open 240 days per year, although it may be more if the practice is accessible on weekends or fewer if the practice is owned by a physician who takes leave. Time is crucial: If the practice in the example were open 365 days per year, 8.52 patients would be needed per day; if the practice was open 240 days per year, that number rises to 12.96; if the practice is open four days a week and the physician's schedule allowed for six weeks of leave per year, 16.55 patients per day would be needed to breakeven.

---

[5] A term for the denominator—revenue per encounter minus variable costs per encounter—is *unit contribution margin*. *Revenue* is defined as NPSR.

The data regarding patient volumes reflect patients who arrive at the practice. Otherwise, the revenue is not received, nor are the variable costs expended. For practical purposes, the breakeven volume is often translated into daily scheduled patient volume. In other words, how many patients need to be scheduled per day to achieve the breakeven volume point?

To calculate the scheduled patient volume, it is important to identify the scheduled-but-not-arrived (SBNA) rate. This rate accounts for the difference between the patients who are scheduled—and the subset of patients who show for their appointments. The SBNA may range from 10% to 25% and can be as high as 50%. To account for the SBNA, take the patient volume needed to breakeven and divide by one minus the SBNA. For the practice in which the physician worked four days a week and took six weeks of leave, 22.1 [16.55/(1 − .25)] would be the volume of patients scheduled per day needed for the practice to break even if the SBNA is 25%. In performing any of these calculations related to breakeven, it is important to recognize that the number must be rounded up as one cannot have a "0.1" encounter. Therefore, to achieve the established goal, in this example, 23 patient visit slots should be incorporated into the schedule.

This basic formula offers significant utility in an ambulatory practice. If a clinician desires a higher income, for example, the additional compensation can be added to the numerator. The breakeven volume point would then be recalculated, and the physician would be consulted to determine if the new volume is achievable. The formula may also be used to model the impact of lower or higher costs, increases or decreases to revenue, changes to time, and so forth. Alternatively, it may be used as a basis for more sophisticated financial models.

It is critical to recognize that volume may not always drive performance in the ambulatory setting; therefore, it is necessary to consider other factors if the practice has pivoted into non-volume-based reimbursement schemes. In that regard, the breakeven analysis should be used exclusively for the FFS side of the business—or altered to account for other factors such as risk.

Clinician Compensation Plans

One of the unique challenges for ambulatory practices is to design a compensation plan for clinicians that is consistent with the mission and culture, as well as financial realities of the practice. Compensation plans also differ based on whether the practice is physician-owned or employed by a third party such as a hospital. Furthermore, the plan may account for differences in earning potential and resource needs based on specialty; this is particularly the case for a practice that maintains more than one specialty (i.e., a multispecialty practice) or a single specialty with several subspecialties. Finally, the plan must be constructed in a manner that is compliant with all laws and regulations.

Practices may negotiate annual salary levels with clinicians or pay each physician an equal share of the revenue remaining once practice costs are paid. However, most ambulatory practices deploy compensation plans that pay variable levels to clinicians based on their production and/or performance. A popular model is to combine both negotiated and variable components, such as a base salary tied to well-defined production and performance expectations, with opportunities to earn additional variable compensation above this base level if specific targets and goals are achieved.

Two key components of clinician compensation plan architectures are (1) the treatment of revenue and (2) the treatment of costs. Each ambulatory practice defines the type of revenue to be included for compensation plan purposes and the performance metrics used to calculate a clinician's revenue contribution. Each practice also determines the costs that are to be charged to physicians. Rarely are two compensation plans alike as there are myriad ways to allocate revenue and costs.

Revenue Treatment

The treatment of revenue for compensation plan purposes may be based on production alone or a combination of production and performance indicators. When designing a compensation plan based on production, what to measure and how to measure production must be determined. For example, production may be based on net professional services revenue generated by the clinician, panel size and panel acuity, number and type of patient encounters, the work relative value unit (WRVU; the component of RVU that relates directly to clinician work effort), some other unit, or a combination of elements. The practice must also detail how other revenue will be treated for compensation planning purposes, such as how to measure and distribute ancillary revenue, hospital directorship stipends, clinical research salaries, and expert witness fees. The method to link compensation and production must also be determined; will the compensation be directly linked, such as a set percentage of net collections or a fixed dollar amount per WRVU, or will the methodology involve more indirect methods, such as targeted ranges and thresholds that must be met? If multiple production measures are used in the compensation plan, they are typically weighted. For example, if the practice elects to employ two production areas for clinician compensation—net collections and WRVUs—it may determine that 70% of the production is to be based on net collections and 30% on WRVUs or some other factor weighting.

When designing a compensation plan that includes *both* production and performance indicators, not only must the production measures as outlined earlier, but also the additional performance measures that will be used for compensation purposes, be determined. For example, an ambulatory practice may decide that clinicians should receive additional compensation for providing extraordinary patient service. If so, decisions as to how to measure service are needed. As an example, if a patient satisfaction instrument is used for this purpose, which patient experience scores are to be used? Do clinicians need to reach a specific threshold, above which their service is deemed extraordinary, or are clinicians to be ranked based on their scores? What dollar value is to be assigned to the service element for compensation planning purposes? As another example, a practice may decide that clinicians should be held accountable for achieving quality metrics for their patient cohorts, such as diabetes screening rates, mammography rates, hospital readmission rates, or surgical outcomes. If so, the compensation plan outlines which metrics to be used and how these will be quantified for compensation planning purposes.

Once the production and performance metrics are identified and measured, the weighting of each of the factors for compensation purposes must be identified. For example, production measures may account for 60% of the revenue assigned with performance measures accounting for 40%, or some other ratio may be applied. These issues are significant and considerable attention by clinicians and practice leaders are required to develop a plan that is legally compliant, fiscally responsible, and one that the clinicians generally believe to be fair and equitable.

Cost Treatment

The compensation plans also differ in the treatment of direct and indirect costs associated with the ambulatory practice. Some practices do not allocate practice costs to clinicians, paying them based on production alone. As an example, a set dollar value for each WRVU is paid with no direct assignment of costs to the clinician. In this example, financial modeling is used to determine the dollars per WRVU that is paid to ensure sufficient revenue to cover practice costs. Others will consider practice costs to be shared among the clinicians, with each clinician held financially responsible for their equal share of the costs. Still, other ambulatory practices perform detailed cost accounting and define the specific costs that are to be shared at the practice level, such as rent, utilities, and general administrative costs, with other costs directly assigned by clinician, such as the salary and benefits of clinical support staff and variable costs associated with patient visit supplies. Consistent with the revenue treatment decisions, the cost treatment of compensation plans involves considerable planning, forecasting, discussion, and debate within the ambulatory practice.

Regardless of the revenue and cost treatment specifically defined by each ambulatory practice, common elements of optimal clinician compensation plan architectures include the following:

- Link to the practice's mission, vision, and goals
- Transparent and understandable plan
- Well-defined goals and expectations
- Fiscally aligned with the practice
- Legally compliant

Physician compensation plans are often considered ideal when they are considered by clinicians to be "equally unfair." The legal compliance issue is critical. Several legal elements impact clinician compensation plan architectures; most ambulatory practices consult with a healthcare attorney when they design or revise their clinical compensation plan. For example, the Stark self-referral law and the federal anti-kickback statute govern federal healthcare programs including Medicare and Medicaid. There are also state law provisions, as well as requirements related to the federal tax code and tax-exempt organizations. These factors impact the methodology that can be used in ambulatory practices to determine the amount of compensation that can be paid to clinicians. In addition to these factors, the status of the clinician as a partner or employee, as well as the specialty, may also constitute important considerations.

Overhead

An often-cited performance measure for an ambulatory practice is its overhead rate. The overhead rate is a measure of a practice's ability to use operating expenses to leverage its revenue-generating assets—clinicians. The overhead rate is determined by dividing operating expenses by NPSR, as noted by the following formula:

$$(\text{total operating costs [fixed + variable]} \div \text{NPSR})$$
$$\times\, 100 = \text{overhead rate (\%)}$$

For example, Rheumatology Associates calculated its total operating costs at $456,955 and its NPSR at $985,001. Using the overhead-rate formula, the overhead rate is 46.39%. For every dollar earned or collected by the practice, $0.46 is spent on overhead costs.

The higher the rate, the less there is to contribute to profitability. The lower the rate, the more the ambulatory practice profits. Profitability may equate to physician compensation for an independent, physician-owned ambulatory practice; it may, instead, mean the practice's financial contribution to its owner. Of course, profit may also be diverted to serve as capital for future investments.

Ambulatory practices that feature surgeons or proceduralists naturally have a lower overhead rate. This may not mean that the surgery practice is spending less than the primary care physician as the overhead rate depends on the numerator (costs) as well as the denominator (revenue). A practice that performs surgeries or procedures typically generates more revenue than a primary care practice, but it also has a portion of its personnel cost born by the facility at which it performs the surgeries or procedures. For example, a surgeon may perform a procedure in a hospital operating room (OR). The OR is distinct from the ambulatory practice where the surgeon holds their office hours. Often, the patient—if ambulant—is seen in the practice before and after the surgery. The practice does not cover the costs of the personnel or the supplies, equipment, or other expenses in the OR

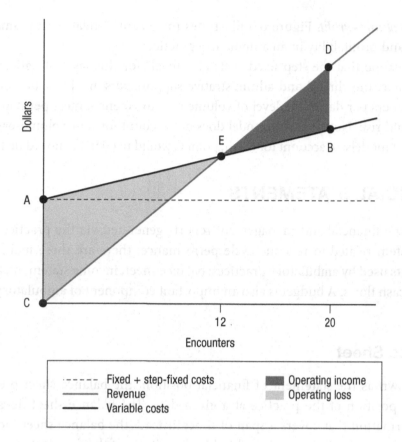

FIGURE 6.6 Cost–volume–profit visualization.

A, Fixed costs + step-fixed costs at 0 encounters per day; B, Total costs (variable + fixed; step-fixed) at 20 encounters per day; C, Revenue at 0 encounters per day; D, Revenue at 20 encounters per day; E, Breakeven point (revenue at 12 encounters per day equals the total costs at 12 encounters per day)

provided by the facility; the facility bills and collects for those separately. The surgeon's revenue, however, is booked to the practice, thus deflating the overhead rate accordingly.

A surgery practice may have an overhead rate of 30%, while the overhead rate of a primary care practice may exceed 60%. The wide difference between the surgery practice and the primary care practice may be based on how costs are allocated within an ambulatory practice. Therefore, one of the key aspects of financial management for an ambulatory practice is the methodology related to cost allocation. Of import, revenue impacts the overhead rate. If a practice narrows its focus to cost reduction without understanding the impact on revenue, the overhead rate may be unchanged or, worse, even higher. Because the overhead rate is a ratio of costs to revenue, if revenue (the denominator) is higher, then the rate falls. Many ambulatory practices discover this strategy to be the key to the financial management of an ambulatory practice: leverage existing resources to produce more value.

Cost–Volume–Profit. Figure 6.6 illustrates the essential relationship among cost, volume, and profitability in an ambulatory practice.

Let's assume that the step-fixed costs are "fixed" for this level of patient volume. For example, the clinical and administrative support personnel remain constant for 25 encounters per day; if the level of volume rose to 50 encounters per day, the fixed costs would rise. Note that this model does not account for non-volume-based reimbursement models; to account for them, point C would need to be moved up the *x*-axis.

FINANCIAL STATEMENTS

Beyond the financial and management reports generated via the practice management system related to revenue cycle performance, there are three main financial statements used by ambulatory practices: balance sheet, income statement, and statement of cash flows. A budget is also an important component of ambulatory practice finances.

Balance Sheet

Also known as the statement of financial position, the balance sheet presents the financial position of the practice at a given date. The balance sheet does not display information that covers a span of time; instead, the balance sheet includes the practice's assets, liabilities, and stockholders' equity as of the final instant of the date shown in its heading (December 31, 20XX, January 31, 20XX, June 30, 20XX, etc.). The following formula summarizes what a balance sheet shows: ASSETS = LIABILITIES + SHAREHOLDERS' EQUITY. Why the term *balance*? The practice's assets must equal, or "balance," the sum of the liabilities and shareholders' equity.

Income Statement

Also known as a profit and loss statement, this statement reports the practice's financial performance in terms of profit over time, such as a month, quarter, or year. Incorporating revenue, expenses, gains, and losses, the income statement demonstrates how much money the practice will make after paying all expenses that have been accrued during the period. Ideally, the statement displays dollars, as well as percentages for each revenue and expense line item, and compares them against historical data and budget amounts. Why the term *income*? After subtracting expenses, the remainder of revenues constitute the practice's income, also referred to as profit. However, do not be surprised if there is no "profit" on the practice's income statement. For independent practices, the physician owners receive salaries (and bonuses) from the practice, often drawing all the profit out to steer clear of double taxation. Accordingly, a practice's income statement may have no profit, thus requiring consideration of compensation and benefits to determine how well the practice is performing financially as a business. The structure of the practice is a vital consideration as different organizational arrangements vary in their tax advantages. Consultation with an accountant familiar with the tax implications of organizational structures is of importance for ambulatory practices.

Statement of Cash Flows

The statement of cash flows reports the movement in cash and bank balances over a period of time. Featuring operating, investing, and financing activities, this report shows a practice's sources and uses of cash for a particular period. Why the term *cash flow*? The statement of cash flow demonstrates the movement of cash—in and out—during the reporting period, which typically coincides with the balance sheet and income statement.

In summary, while each financial statement is presented separately, they are all interrelated. The changes in assets and liabilities that may be seen on the balance sheet are accounted for in the revenues and expenses on the income statement, for example. No single financial statement reveals the complete story; combined, however, these statements provide powerful information about the oversight, management, and decision-making for an ambulatory practice.

Budget

Creating and maintaining a budget provides a solid foundation to manage the finances of an ambulatory practice using a disciplined approach. Budgets are commonly formulated on an annual basis, aligning with the calendar or fiscal year. Several months before the commencement of the year, the manager or management team develops estimates of revenue and expenses.

Ideally, the budget is more granular than simply an estimate of revenue and expenses. The budgeted revenue includes a thoughtful approach to an estimate that accounts for services, volume, coding, expected reimbursement from payers, receivables management, payer mix, and place of service. Anticipated shifts in any of these categories would impact the budgeted revenue; this may include changes to reimbursement models, laws or regulations, or market dynamics such as population growth.

From a cost perspective, the budgeted costs are presented in categories. The estimated cost associated with each major expenditure, personnel, information technology, and so forth are reported. Many ambulatory practices maintain a standard chart of accounts to allow for historical tracking and trending of expenditures. The expenses associated with marketing, for example, would be grouped and reported together. The practice could, therefore, measure and monitor actual marketing expenses against the budget—as well as compare this to the year prior's marketing expenses.

As the year begins, the budget provides a framework for financial expectations. Actual expenses are reported in categories aligned with the budget. A budget never solves a financial crisis; however, it allows stakeholders to be forewarned. For example, perhaps the revenue is not meeting expectations. Instead of waiting until the end of the year to find out that the physician must liquidate the practice's bank account just to make payroll, dips in revenues or boosts in expenses throughout the year are identified, and interventions can be formulated and deployed.

CONCLUSION

The financial management of an ambulatory practice extends beyond the typical steps by business enterprises to manage revenue, expenses, and profits. The revenue cycle—consisting of all the steps required to document, bill, and collect for a clinical service—is complex, requiring personnel with exacting skill sets to practice due diligence to ensure ideal financial performance. Revenue optimization must be matched by a thoughtful approach to expense management, enabling the ambulatory practice to maximize its profits. These efforts can be supported by financial statements, as well as a budget to sustain a practice's journey to financial success.

DISCUSSION QUESTIONS

1. Why was it problematic that historically clinicians would simply record the services they performed?

2. Why are physician compensation plans often considered ideal when they are considered by clinicians to be "equally unfair"?

3. Why is the term *cash flow* used in one of the three main financial statements used by ambulatory practices?

4. What is an example of a variable cost in an ambulatory practice?

REFERENCES

American Medical Association. (2021). *CPT® 2021*.

Centers for Medicare and Medicaid Services. (2019, October). *Place of service codes for professional claims database*. https://www.cms.gov/Medicare/Coding/place-of-service-codes/Place_of_Service_Code_Set

Centers for Medicare and Medicaid Services. (n.d.). *How to use the searchable Medicare physician fee schedule*. https://www.cms.gov/files/document/2020-physician-fee-schedule-guide.pdf

Medicare Payment Advisory Commission. (2016, October). *Outpatient hospital services payment system*. http://www.medpac.gov/docs/default-source/payment-basics/medpac_payment_basics_16_opd_final.pdf

Washington Publishing Company. (n.d.). *Claim adjustment reason codes.* https://x12.org/codes/claim-adjustment-reason-codes

World Health Organization. (n.d.). *International Statistical Classification of Diseases and Related Health Problems (ICD).* https://www.who.int/standards/classifications/classification-of-diseases

HUMAN RESOURCES

LEARNING OBJECTIVES

1. Understand the key roles of clinicians, clinical support personnel, and administrative support personnel and how they work collaboratively in an ambulatory practice

2. Identify regulatory considerations that influence the management of ambulatory practice personnel

3. Describe trends and concepts developed to support and optimize the ambulatory care workforce

KEY TERMS

Organizational Chart

Advanced Practice Provider

Benchmarks

Patient Panel

Scope of Practice

Care Team

Top of License

Telework

INTRODUCTION

The workforce of an ambulatory practice has no singular definition. Employees differ based on the composition of the practice. The labor pool may change based on the practice's evolution: A new procedure may prompt the need for new personnel, an alteration in the **scope of practice** laws may result in a change of credentials required for a position, or a new employee may be needed to support the practice's growth. Human resources in an ambulatory practice is a complex, ever-changing topic. Because people formulate the basis of the practice's delivery of care—and how that care is delivered—the management of human resources in an ambulatory practice is of utmost importance.

PERSONNEL

The volume and type of personnel in an ambulatory practice vary based on the nature of the specialty, the services delivered, the ownership, and the size of the practice. Specialty practices with ancillary services, such as imaging or laboratories, will have more personnel than practices than those offering a more limited scope. Hospital- or health system-owned practices may be supported by administrative staff based in hospital departments, such as information technology (IT), accounting, and facility maintenance, rather than have dedicated personnel deployed to these functions. Larger practices may have formal organizational structures with employees not only devoted to clinical service support but also accompanied by an administrative infrastructure consistent with their size, scope, and complexity.

All practices, regardless of specialty, services, ownership, and size, have clinicians and a support team of personnel devoted to clinical and administrative work functions. These employees are typically supported by one or more directors, managers, and/or supervisors to provide leadership and direction to the team.

Clinicians

An ambulatory practice may have one—or more—physicians. Practices with one physician are commonly referred to as "solo" practices. Practices with more than one physician are typically referred to as "group" practices. Among medical practices, 14% of physicians were represented in solo practices in 2020, while the remaining percentage of physicians worked in group practices. The percentage of physicians in practices with 50 or more physicians was 17.2% in 2020 (American Medical Association [AMA], 2021). In states that allow the organization of a practice by a nonphysician, ambulatory practices may also be owned and operated by **advanced practice providers** or other healthcare professionals.

The physicians working in ambulatory practices offer primary care, medical specialty, surgical specialty, or ancillary specialty services consistent with their training. The practices may also have one or more advanced practice providers, including physician assistants, nurse practitioners, certified nurse midwives, or one of a multitude of other practitioners. Together, the physicians and advanced practice providers are known as "clinicians," and they may also be accompanied by one or more healthcare professionals who provide care, support, education, and outreach to patients.

The clinician staffing of ambulatory practices differs based on specialty, consistent with the services that specialty provides. Within a specified specialty, however, there are common staffing patterns. for example, an otolaryngology practice may have an otolaryngologist, an audiologist, and a physician assistant; an endocrinology practice may have an endocrinologist, a certified diabetic educator, and a clinical nurse specialist; a student health practice may have a family medicine physician and a nurse practitioner;

and an orthopedic practice may have an orthopedic surgeon and a physical therapist. The clinicians in these practices may travel to the hospital to perform or assist in surgery, consult on patients in the hospital or other facility, or remain exclusively in the ambulatory setting. Other ambulatory practice settings, such as an ambulatory surgery center, may have a dedicated management and support team, with clinicians contracting to use the space to perform ambulatory procedures and surgeries.

Advanced practice providers play an essential role in ambulatory practices. Table 7.1 displays the number and mix of clinicians billing under the Medicare Physician Fee Schedule (PFS). Although this incorporates all care settings, the data demonstrate the growth of advanced practice providers as clinicians.

TABLE 7.1 Number of Clinicians Billing Under the Medicare Physician Fee Schedule, 2014–2019

	2014	2015	2016	2017	2018	2019
	# (IN THOUSANDS)					
PHYSICIANS, PRIMARY CARE SPECIALTIES	141	141	141	140	139	139
PHYSICIANS, OTHER SPECIALTIES	432	439	447	455	461	468
APRNS AND PAS	161	178	198	218	237	258
OTHER PRACTITIONERS	156	161	167	172	178	184
TOTAL	890	919	952	985	1015	1048
	# PER 1,000 BENEFICIARIES					
PHYSICIANS, PRIMARY CARE SPECIALTIES	2.9	2.8	2.7	2.6	2.5	2.5
PHYSICIANS, OTHER SPECIALTIES	8.8	8.7	8.6	8.5	8.4	8.3
APRNS AND PAS	3.2	3.5	3.8	4.1	4.3	4.6
OTHER PRACTITIONERS	3.2	3.2	3.2	3.2	3.2	3.3
TOTAL	18.0	18.1	18.3	18.4	18.5	18.7

SOURCE: Medicare Payment Advisory Commission. (2021, March). *Report to the Congress: Medicare payment policyC* (p. 109).

NOTE: Primary care specialties" include family medicine, internal medicine, pediatric medicine, and geriatric medicine, with an adjustment to exclude hospitalists. Hospitalists are counted in "other specialties." "Other practitioners" include clinicians such as physical therapists, psychologists, social workers, and podiatrists. The number of clinicians shown in this table includes only those with a caseload of more than 15 beneficiaries in the year. Beneficiary counts used to calculate clinicians per 1,000 beneficiaries include those enrolled in traditional Medicare Part B and those in Medicare Advantage, based on the assumption that clinicians generally furnish services to beneficiaries in both programs. Numbers exclude nonperson providers such as clinical laboratories and independent diagnostic testing facilities. Components may not sum to totals due to rounding.

APRN, advanced practice registered nurse; PA, physician assistant

The number and type of clinicians in an ambulatory practice are typically determined based on community need, internal and external **benchmarks**, the regulatory environment, and reimbursement opportunity as further described later. There are also considerations based on the size and type of the facility, as well as staffing.

Community Need

Clinician volume and type are often dictated and aligned with the population of patients in the community. Data regarding the volume of encounters by specialty based on population density are available from the National Ambulatory Medical Care Survey (NAMCS) and the National Hospital Ambulatory Medical Care Survey (NHAMCS), studies administered by the National Center for Health Statistics under the Centers for Disease Control and Prevention. Table 7.2 provides national physician office and hospital outpatient visit data annually for available years. These data assist in determining the appropriate volume and type of clinicians required to meet patient demand.

Specific community needs for patient services and patient access may also dictate the clinician practice size, regardless of the volume of patients. If the actual or predicted patient volume does not support the practice from a business perspective, financial subsidies may be available from an external entity to permit a practice to size itself beyond what is needed simply to meet patient volume demand. Before entering a formal relationship featuring financial support, the parties should consult an attorney familiar with healthcare law, as there are legal issues that may impact such a relationship.

The constitution of the "community" of a practice, which also may be considered the "market" in the context of analyzing the catchment area for a clinician, depends on the practice specialty as well as geography. For example, a pediatric neurooncologist may consider its community a multistate area given its specialization, while a pediatrician may serve families within a five-mile radius of the practice. Typically, primary care is offered locally via an ambulatory practice that has a physical location in the community; alternatively, patients may seek services provided by a clinician practicing out of a retailer. The services may be offered via telemedicine, whereby local clinicians provide care via a remote platform that allows the patient to remain at home. Alternatively, the services may be offered by practicing clinicians across the country via telemedicine. Specialty practices, including medical specialties and surgical specialties, may be regionally distributed. The practice may feature clinicians practicing in a community-based practice location owned by the physicians or have a hospital-employed team situated in a multidisciplinary ambulatory practice adjacent to the inpatient bed tower. Specialists, too, may rely on a virtual platform particularly for initial consultations and post-surgical care. Primary care and specialty practices may be joined by other ambulatory practices—a community health center may be sited in the locale, the local public health

TABLE 7.2 Annual Physician Office and Hospital Outpatient Visits in the United States, 1973–2016

YEAR	PHYSICIAN OFFICE VISITS[a] (MILLIONS)	PHYSICIAN OFFICE VISIT RATE (PER PERSON)	HOSPITAL OUTPATIENT VISITS[b] (THOUSANDS)	HOSPITAL OUTPATIENT VISIT RATE (PER 100 PERSONS)
1973	644.9	3.1		
1974	577.8			
1975	567.6	2.7		
1976	588.3	2.8		
1977	570	2.7		
1978	584.5	2.8		
1979	556.3	2.6		
1980	575.7	2.7		
1981	585.2	2.6		
1982				
1983				
1984				
1985	636.4	2.7		
1986				
1987				
1988				
1989	692.7	2.8		
1990	704.6	2.9		
1991	669.7	2.7		
1992	762	3	56.6	22.5
1993	717.2	2.8	62.5	24.6
1994	681.5	2.6	66.3	25.6
1995	697.1	2.7	67.2	25.7
1996	734.5	2.8	67.2	25.4
1997	787.4	3.0	77.0	28.9
1998	829.3	3.1	75.4	28

(continued)

TABLE 7.2 Annual Physician Office and Hospital Outpatient Visits in the United States, 1973–2016 (*Continued*)

YEAR	PHYSICIAN OFFICE VISITS[a] (MILLIONS)	PHYSICIAN OFFICE VISIT RATE (PER PERSON)	HOSPITAL OUTPATIENT VISITS[b] (THOUSANDS)	HOSPITAL OUTPATIENT VISIT RATE (PER 100 PERSONS)
1999	756.7	2.785	84.6	31.1
2000	823.5	3.004	83.3	30.4
2001	880.5	3.144	83.7	29.9
2002	890	3.144	83.3	29.4
2003	906	3.173	94.6	33.1
2004	910.9	3.159	85	29.5
2005	963.6	3.31	90.4	31
2006	902	3.066	102.2	34.7
2007	994.3	3.356	88.9	30
2008	956.0	3.201	109.9	36.8
2009	1037.8	3.441	96.1	31.9
2010	1008.8	3.322	100.7	33.2
2011	987.0	3.222	125.7	41
2012	928.6	3.008	-	-
2013	922.6	2.967	-	-
2014	884.7	2.8	-	-
2015	990.8	3.133	-	-
2016	883.7	2.779	-	-

NOTE: Physician office visit data retrieved from the NAMCS conducted annually beginning 1973; hospital outpatient visit data retrieved from NHAMCS conducted annually beginning 1992; NHAMCS data from 2012 to 2016 not released due to quality assurance issues.

[a]Includes patient visits to nonfederal, office-based physicians

[b]Includes patient visits to outpatient departments of nonfederal, short-stay hospitals

SOURCE: NAMCS/NHAMCS data was retrieved from summary reports published by the Centers for Disease Control and Prevention, National Center for Health Statistics. *Advance data from vital and health statistics.* https://www.cdc.gov/nchs/products/ad.htm. All material appearing in this report is in the public domain.

department may offer immunizations, or a mobile clinic may provide screening exams. As the nature of ambulatory practices differs, so, too, do the communities they serve.

One will often hear the term *local primary care and regional specialty care* to depict the geographic distribution of ambulatory practices, although technology is rapidly changing the traditional brick-and-mortar delivery of ambulatory care.

Internal Benchmarks

Ambulatory practices may use internal benchmarks such as practice-level scheduling data to drive decisions about clinician capacity management. If, for example, new patient appointments are increasingly stretching weeks or months in the future, the practice may commence an assessment of whether a new clinician is needed to meet growing patient demand. Referral data are also valuable in the case of a specialty practice. If referrals are queuing without the ability to accommodate them in a timely manner, this may prompt further reevaluation of the current clinician capacity. The same consideration is given when clinicians announce their departure or retirement, or an unforeseen event triggers the loss of a clinician. Practices use these inputs to determine whether the departing clinician should be replaced and, if so, the type of clinician that is needed: a physician, advanced practice provider, or another healthcare professional. Studying and assessing demand based on internal data is often overlooked by practices but offers exceptional insight into the issue of ascertaining clinician staffing.

External Benchmarks

Determinations regarding the number and type of clinicians for a specific ambulatory practice can be enhanced by utilizing productivity benchmark data available from professional associations, specialty societies, and vendors. Survey benchmark data are typically published annually from professional associations, but specialty societies and vendors will often query their members and share data in a timelier manner. For example, a specialty society may gather responses from its members that daily patient visit volumes average 25 patients per day. From these data, a practice in that specialty can use that benchmark to validate its clinicians volumes. A practice in the specialty may see an average of 150 patients per day. Given the average visit volume of 25 patients per day per clinician, this suggests the need for 6.00 full-time-equivalent (FTE) clinicians to meet the daily patient visit volume (calculated as 150 divided by 25). Another measure is work relative value units, which better account for varying work complexities.

Patient panel benchmarks may also be useful in primary care when determining the appropriate clinician volume for an ambulatory practice. The nature of primary care dictates a relationship with the patient over time, and there are often activities that occur between the clinician–patient visit. The management of preventive services, counseling and coordination of care, and triage and advice are the hallmark of primary care. As such, the size of a primary care practice need not be measured by the number of patients seen per day but rather by the total number of patients who are actively cared for. Typically measured in a three-year term, a patient panel is defined as the number of unique patients (in contrast to visits) seen during this period. As an example, a specialty association may report a median of 3,000 unique patients for their specialty. For an ambulatory practice with 15,000 patients, this would suggest the need for 5.00 FTE clinicians (calculated as 15,000 divided by 3,000). The optimal panel size may be adjusted based on patient-level characteristics such as gender, payer, and age. For example, infants and senior patients generally demand more services, so the size of a patient panel of very young and very aged patients may be lower than the size of a patient panel comprised of healthy adults aged 20 to 50 years old. There may also be further adjustments to the patient panel size based on various social determinants of health. Table 7.3 offers a calculated panel weighting for age, gender, and insurance categories as determined by an observational study of 27 primary care clinics that served more than 150,000 patients.

TABLE 7.3 Calculated Panel Weighting for Age, Gender, and Insurance Categories

AGE (IN YEARS)	INSURANCE	MALES WEIGHT	FEMALES WEIGHT
0–3	Medicare	1.00	1.00
	Medicaid	1.51	1.44
	Other	1.64	1.55
4–14	Medicare	1.00	2.62
	Medicaid	0.85	0.78
	Other	0.84	0.82
15–39	Medicare	1.15	1.82
	Medicaid	0.69	1.20
	Other	0.53	0.81
40–59	Medicare	1.65	2.22
	Medicaid	1.13	1.45
	Other	0.80	1.00
60–74	Medicare	1.52	1.71
	Medicaid	1.42	1.57
	Other	1.12	1.21
>75	Medicare	1.89	1.98
	Medicaid	1.04	1.71
	Other	1.33	1.09

SOURCE: Kamnetz, S., Trowbridge, E., Lochner, J., Koslov, S., & Pandhi, N. (2018). A simple framework for weighting panels across primary care disciplines: Findings from a large US multidisciplinary group practice. *Quality Management in Health Care, 27*(4), 187. https://doi.org/10.1097/QMH.0000000000000190

NOTE: Other category includes all other payers (i.e., health maintenance organizations, commercial insurance companies, and other insurers). Dual-eligible beneficiaries were assigned to their primary insurance.

Beyond these benchmarks that relate the number of clinicians to the work or patient volume, it is important to remember that healthcare is a service industry in which a high degree of quality is expected and demanded. Benchmarks may need to be revised based on periodic review of service provisions to ensure that high-quality care and outcomes are achieved.

Regulatory Environment

An essential consideration for human resources in an ambulatory practice relates to the regulatory environment. Healthcare professionals have a designated scope of practice that varies by state. The American Nursing Association (n.d.) defines the scope of practice as "the services that a qualified health professional is deemed competent to perform and permitted to undertake—in keeping with the terms of their professional license." In one state, for example, a nurse practitioner may prescribe medications as an independent practitioner, while the adjacent state's declared scope of practice may prohibit that action. In addition to work tasks, the state may also dictate supervision requirements. One state may require a physician to countersign the records of every patient seen and treated by a nurse practitioner; the adjacent state may only require a onetime practice agreement between all parties. These regulations extend to all clinical personnel, which is also dictated by the given state's scope of practice. Because this scope of practice may involve tasks that are routinely performed in the ambulatory practice, such as injections, it is crucial to understand any scope of practice restrictions that are applicable for the practice.

Other stakeholders may play a role related to the regulatory environment. The practice may have credentialing requirements—for example, a hospital-owned ambulatory surgery center may require an application and approval process administered by the hospital in order to practice. Malpractice carriers may also be a factor; coverage may not be available to all clinicians or support personnel, which may influence determinations related to staffing.

Reimbursement

Reimbursement may play a role in the clinical staffing pattern in an ambulatory practice, as insurance companies may not provide coverage of the services rendered by some clinician types. This may include, for example, certified nurse specialists providing services as independent clinicians. Even though the certified nurse specialist may be able to perform the service per state law, the insurance company may not agree to pay for it. In another scenario, an ambulatory practice may be organized and enrolled as a hospital outpatient clinic; it may, therefore, not be able to bill separately for professional services provided by certain hospital-employed, nonphysician clinicians. The services of these clinicians may be included in the reimbursement for the facility but not represent a separate billable service.

In sum, many factors impact clinician staffing in an ambulatory practice: community need; patient volume and panel size, factors that may be compared to industry benchmarks; regulations; malpractice coverage; and reimbursement. The facility itself, as well as trained staff to support the clinician, are also important considerations. Even if all these factors are favorable, a clinician who fits the needs of the practice must be proximal, available, and willing to serve as a clinician in the practice.

Clinical Support Personnel

Almost half of the physician's workday, on average, is spent outside of the patient encounter conducting nonclinical, administrative tasks (Gottschalk & Flock, 2005). It is vital that physicians have a support team to delegate work consistent with licensure and scope of practice. Clinical support personnel play an important role in ensuring efficient, effective, and reliably consistent clinical practice and quality outcomes.

Much like clinicians, the clinical support personnel vary in volume and type. Clinical support personnel include registered nurses (RNs), licensed practical nurses (LPNs) and licensed vocational nurses (LVNs, a title used in California and Texas in place of LPN), and medical assistants (MAs) or certified medical assistants (CMAs). Based on the specialty of the ambulatory practice and its breadth of services, there may be additional clinical support that is necessary, such as radiology technicians and clinical laboratory personnel. In general, clinicians are a provider type who can bill for their services, while clinical support personnel serve in nonbillable support roles. There are some exceptions, however, such as specific nurse visits that may be billed in certain ambulatory settings.

Scope-of-practice laws that vary by state are integral to clinical personnel staffing, just as they are relevant for clinicians. States that do not allow MAs to render injections, for example, influence staffing determinations particularly when the need for that task is high. Consider, for example, a pediatrics practice that provides vaccinations. When clinical personnel are prohibited from performing injections due to state law, the responsibility must be shifted to another party. The tasks are transferred to the physician or advanced practice providers out of legal necessity. Such laws have a significant impact on the workflow and the number of clinicians needed in the practice. Therefore, clinical personnel requirements are dictated by the type of services to be provided, and the scope of practice granted these personnel based on state law.

Similar to the treatment of clinicians, the scope of practice for support personnel may further be defined based on the requirements of the facility and the malpractice carrier. A hospital, for example, may permit nursing staff to conduct specific aspects of wound care, while others may assign this role to advanced practice providers.

In addition to the *type* of clinical personnel, the *number* of clinical personnel is an important consideration for ambulatory practices. Benchmark data that involves staffing based on the number of clinicians supported may be available from professional associations, specialty societies, and vendors. These "staff per FTE physician" or "staff per FTE provider" (to include both physicians and nonphysician clinicians) ratios, however, do not account for work volume. As an example, if a practice adopts a static staffing model to assign one full-time RN to each physician, regardless of whether a physician sees eight or 38 patients per day, the practice will not achieve an optimal staffing pattern consistent with the work to be performed. Staffing ratios may be best formulated based on time-and-motion studies and observations related to the type and number of tasks performed by each individual.

The growing proliferation of remote care in recent years requires ambulatory practices to staff for these novel work functions. Preparing for virtual visits, conducting patient outreach, providing support during care transitions, interpreting test data from mobile health devices, and other related tasks expand the work scope of traditional ambulatory practices. Although some practices have attempted to assign current staff with the additional responsibilities of remote care, others have created a staffing model that is separate and distinct from the traditional face-to-face (F2F) visit, with one team dedicated to remote care and another to F2F care. Tasks may be divided between the teams; both the clinical and administrative personnel may be dedicated to remote versus F2F, or alternatively, the clinical personnel only. Exhibit 7.1 presents an example of the division of work for an ambulatory practice that offers remote visits.

Administrative Support Personnel

The administrative support personnel in an ambulatory practice handle the non-clinical tasks required of a practice. These include assisting the patient flow process as well as the infrastructure for communications, IT, revenue cycle, finance and accounting, human resources, and facilities and maintenance. The general work functions and responsibilities typically assigned to core personnel are outlined in

EXHIBIT 7.1 CARE MANAGEMENT TEAM TASKS: VIRTUAL AND FACE-TO-FACE

Virtual Care Management Team Tasks	Face-to-Face Care Management Team Tasks
Pre-encounter scrub	Clinical intake and rooming
Virtual patient communication	Clinical support
Care monitoring	Medication preparation; administration
Virtual clinical intake and rooming	Training, education, and instructions
Result communication	Orders; referrals for care

the following sections. This should not be considered an exhaustive list, as the needs of an ambulatory practice may dictate additional staff functions. Responsibilities are typically managed by in-house personnel; however, tasks may be outsourced to a third party or handled by the practice's owner at a corporate level. Furthermore, the practice may rely on contractors or temporary employees.

Patient Flow

Administrative personnel conduct the pre-arrival responsibilities of registration and scheduling as well as the arrival of the patient. They also facilitate the actions recommended by the clinician after the patient's encounter, including referrals, testing, ancillary testing, and other post-encounter tasks.

Communications

Communications personnel manage inbound and outbound phone calls, portal and text messages, chats, and other information transmitted to and from the practice. They also may conduct patient outreach for inter-visit care needs.

Information Technology

IT staff build, install, maintain, and support the practice management and electronic health record system(s) of the practice, as well as the computing needs of both clinicians and staff. IT staff may support one or more other technology systems or solutions deployed by the practice. This team may also initiate and service the practice's hardware, including computers, tablets, kiosks, and other devices.

Revenue Cycle

Front office and business office personnel typically are assigned to specific roles relating to revenue cycle management, including, but not limited to, charge capture, coding, claim submission, account follow-up, payment posting, refunds management, collections, and data management.

Finance and Accounting

Finance and accounting staff manage purchasing, payroll, equipment inventory, investments, capital expenditures, budgeting, refunds, and other associated finance and accounting tasks.

Human Resources

Human resources staff are involved in the recruitment and retention of personnel, compensation, and benefits management. They may also be involved with quality improvement initiatives, such as performance monitoring among clinicians or professional development opportunities among clinical and administrative personnel.

Facilities and Maintenance

Facility management personnel are responsible for any facility-related tasks including the management of utilities, housekeeping, and building repair or construction.

The titles associated with administrative personnel in an ambulatory practice vary. As an example, a common name for the personnel managing the administrative aspects of patient flow is "patient service representatives" (PSRs). However, the same roles may also be referred to as "receptionists", "front office staff", "customer service representatives", "**care team** associates", or other titles. Similarly, administrative personnel assigned to manage the account follow-up tasks in the business office may be referred to as "account follow-up representatives", "billers", "revenue optimization staff", "insurance follow-up representatives", and other associated titles. It is thus important to identify the specific work tasks assigned to administrative personnel rather than rely on titles when seeking to compare and contrast staffing models of an ambulatory practice.

As the practice expands, the functions performed by the administrative personnel become more specific. Instead of a PSR single-handedly managing registration, scheduling, telephones, messages, arrival, and so forth, there is a team dedicated to each functional area or a cluster of functions. For example, a registration team may be formed to handle registration-specific exceptions such as patients with expired coverage, out-of-network patients, and patients who require authorization from their insurance company to be seen. A scheduling team may be dedicated to all incoming calls, messages, chats, texts, and other requests for appointments; alternatively, they may be formulated to accept requests from new patients or referral sources only. Another team may be responsible for processing outbound referrals. Because work functions vary by specialty and type of practice, the composition, size, and duties associated with teams differ. As the practice grows, more people are needed to process tasks, and the functions are organized with more specific tasks in mind. The clustering and organization of tasks allow for targeted recruitment, training, technology, quality assurance, workforce management, and supervision.

Like clinical personnel, there are benchmark data regarding administrative staffing ratios based on the number of clinicians in an ambulatory practice. The challenges related to these ratios not accounting for actual work volume are consistent with that of clinical personnel. Therefore, internal assessment related to the type and scope of work is recommended.

Staff workload ranges for key ambulatory practice positions are presented in Table 7.4; these data may provide a valuable supplement to internal assessments about the ideal type and volume of personnel required for the ambulatory practice.

TABLE 7.4 Daily Employee Workload Ranges

TASK	DAILY WORKLOAD RANGE PER EMPLOYEE	STAFF TYPE ASSOCIATED WITH TASK
FULL REGISTRATION	60 to 80 patients	Patient service representative
MINI-REGISTRATION	80 to 100 patients	Patient service representative
FULL SCHEDULING + REGISTRATION ("SCHEDGISTRATION")	55 to 75 patients	Scheduler
SCHEDULING	50 to 75 appointments	Scheduler
SURGERY SCHEDULING	30 to 40 surgeries	Scheduler
NURSE TRIAGE + ADVICE	60 to 80 patients	Nurse
PRACTICE SERVICES (RETURN VISIT SCHEDULING, VISIT CLOSURE)	50 to 75 patients	Patient service representative
REFERRALS	30 to 50 referrals	Patient service representative
PRIOR AUTHORIZATIONS	30 to 50 authorizations	Patient service representative

NOTE: "Daily" is defined herein as an eight-hour day. The workload ranges depend on the length of the business day, patient population (including the percentage of new versus established), information systems, required data, automation, and work processes used at the practice. To apply these ranges, consider measuring the time it takes for your employees to handle each task, and then apply that transaction time (after applying a downtime factor, typically 70% to 80%, depending on the task) to reach a practice's ideal workload range.

Management

The management structure varies by ambulatory practice; however, there is typically a dedicated manager. The manager may be a clinician or nonclinician, or the practice may be managed by a physician–administrator team of two individuals, with the physician administrator focused on clinical management and the nonphysician administrator focused on managing the business and nonclinical affairs of the practice. These physician–administrator dyads are commonly found in large ambulatory practices. The size of the organization will determine if the practice has a dedicated manager or a manager who splits their time among several sites or practices.

Ambulatory practices maintain a medley of organizational structures. Figures 7.1 through 7.4 outline sample organizational structures, from a solo or small practice to a large ambulatory enterprise embedded in a health system. These are only examples as it is common to find variations of organizational structures based on the size of the practice (to include the number and scale of practice sites); the number and types of clinical services that constitute the practice; the preference of leaders; the training, skills, and experiences of persons engaged in management; and the overall management needs of the practice. The management may also be contracted from a third party.

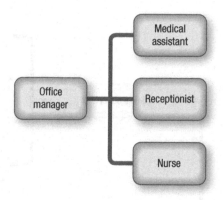

FIGURE 7.1 Small ambulatory practice—sample organizational chart.

As with other administrative roles, the specific title used for the lead administrative officer of the ambulatory practice varies. It may be an office manager, practice manager, practice administrator, vice president of ambulatory care, or chief ambulatory medical officer. Large practices may have a full management team with a chief executive officer, chief financial officer, chief operating officer, and other C-suite executives found in other healthcare organizations. The management team may reside at the corporate level, with each ambulatory practice (or group of practices) assigned a practice manager to provide oversight. In a hospital or health system, the ambulatory practices may reside in a separate division or may report to the hospital's chief operating officer, chief medical officer, or another senior executive. The ambulatory practices related to the service line may report directly to the service line administrator. For example, the ambulatory practices of orthopedics, sports medicine, physiatry, physical and occupational therapy, occupational medicine, and musculoskeletal imaging report to the musculoskeletal service line administrator. Furthermore, the management may be shared, as is common with a dyad of an administrator and a physician leader.

There is no specified career pathway to become a manager of an ambulatory practice; many have training, skills, and education in healthcare and business. Some have a clinical background; others worked in management in an industry with skill sets that overlap those needed to manage an ambulatory practice. Others may have served in support positions but migrated into management when the opportunity arose. Skills, training, and education vary; however, enjoying the complex, constantly changing nature of an ambulatory practice is a consistent theme among managers.

KEY CONSIDERATIONS

Personnel are essential to an ambulatory practice. There are important considerations related to human resources beyond the number, type, and accounting of

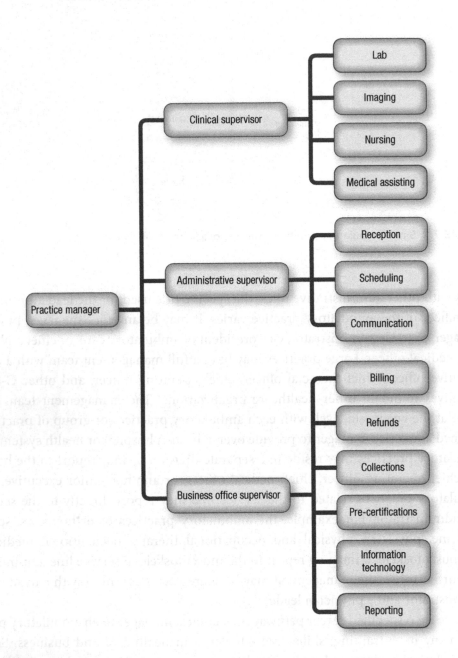

FIGURE 7.2 Midsized ambulatory practice—sample organization chart.

personnel deployed. Human resources concepts important to an ambulatory practice are explored in the following section.

Job Description

There are many benefits from having documented job descriptions for all personnel of an ambulatory practice. First, the job description establishes expectations for the

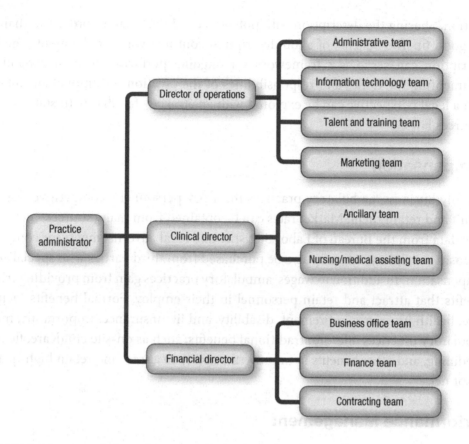

FIGURE 7.3 Large ambulatory practice—sample organizational chart.

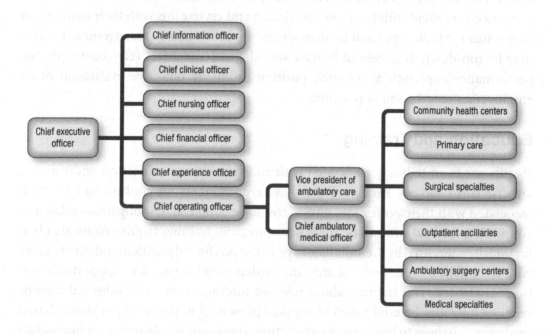

FIGURE 7.4 Hospital-based ambulatory practice—sample organizational chart.

position. Sharing the description with potential candidates can improve the chances of a good fit. The benefits of a job description continue with employment. The job description can serve as a framework for ongoing performance management by documenting the duties and responsibilities of the position. Additional advantages from a legal perspective can be explored with an attorney familiar with state human resources laws.

Compensation

Like any business, ambulatory practices must pay personnel a competitive wage to recruit and retain them. Market rates can be obtained from many sources, including wage data from the Bureau of Labor Statistics and local advertisements for comparable positions. Salary data may also be purchased from third parties who specialize in compensation. In addition to wages, ambulatory practices gain from providing fringe benefits that attract and retain personnel in their employ. Formal benefits include leave, health insurance, retirement, disability, and life insurance. Importantly, many ambulatory practices offer nontraditional benefits, such as on-site childcare, flexible scheduling, and other benefits to improve the ability to attract and retain high-quality personnel.

Performance Management

A formal performance management process is typically used by ambulatory practices on at least an annual basis. Personnel may be asked to self-evaluate their performance consistent with their job description and review this with their manager or supervisor for their input and finalization, or the performance management process may be top-down. It is helpful to have well-defined and effectively communicated performance expectations for each position to ensure objective evaluation of an employee's strengths and opportunities.

Education and Training

Healthcare is an industry associated with constant change; education and training are crucial to success. Personnel may have requirements for continuing education associated with their profession; physicians, for example, have obligations related to continuing medical education. These education and training requirements are often financially supported by the ambulatory practice. As clinical practice guidelines evolve with the publication of new research and evidence, many practices support orientation, discussion, and training about relevant findings. Formal or informal mentor relationships may be established to support personnel in delivering evidence-based medicine. Changes to laws, payer contracting, rules, and regulations may necessitate that personnel receive education and training. Similarly, as the patient flow process changes to more remote and virtual care delivery, personnel must learn new skill sets. Furthermore, ambulatory practices typically offer a combination of in-service, online, and remote training opportunities for personnel to ensure knowledge and skill currency remains consistent with the rapidly changing environment.

TRENDS
Care Team

Given the complexity and work volume inherent to an ambulatory practice, it is essential to work together as a team to care for patients. Teamwork involves communication and collaboration among parties. It may also include a more formal structure wherein personnel are assigned to a specific team that may entail rotating responsibilities. The team may be small—a physician and medical assistant may work together—or may involve multiple parties to include pharmacists, health coaches, and behavioral health specialists, among others.

Teamwork in a healthcare setting is facilitated by key principles, as laid out by researchers Warde et al. (2019) who developed the Conceptual Model of Interprofessional Team Performance. Although the framework was established for a primary care setting, the principles apply to ambulatory practices. Figure 7.5 displays the structural elements that influence the team; the performance domains; the overarching culture of a work environment based on transparency, trust, and relationships; and the expected team outcomes.

This team approach to human resources is widely used in ambulatory practices. This is a result of the complex nature of ambulatory care; patients benefit from accessing the skills and efforts of multiple personnel working in collaboration to manage their care and treatment.

Top of License

The Institute of Medicine (IOM) issued the report *The Future of Nursing: Leading Change, Advancing Health* in 2010 (IOM, 2010). The IOM promulgated the recommendation: "Nurses should practice to the full extent of their education." This suggestion led to extensive efforts in the ambulatory setting related to job delineation for all clinical positions. To address clinical responsibilities, administrative personnel have also been engaged to promote ideal task alignment. The collective initiatives related to leveraging education and training at its fullest extent have emerged using the term *top of license* (TOL). Ambulatory practices have integrated TOL initiatives by reconfiguring tasks as well as personnel. Performing work maximal to education, as well as training, skills, and experience, improves healthcare access (Berry, 2003).

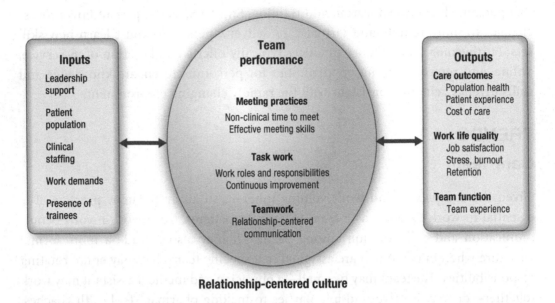

FIGURE 7.5 Conceptual model of care team performance.

SOURCE: Warde, C. M., Giannitrapani, K. F., & Pearson, M. L. (2020). Teaching primary care teamwork: A conceptual model of primary care team performance. *The Clinical Teacher, 17*(3), 250. https://doi.org/10.1111/tct.13037

Telework

Ambulatory practices may permit telework accommodations, as the position allows. The COVID-19 pandemic accelerated this work pathway, with select categories of personnel conducting business and clinical functions from their home or remotely wherever they have the appropriate technology and security measures in place. For example, entire call centers serving as ambulatory scheduling hubs for hospitals or health systems have been transitioned from on-site offices to independent home offices, a migration often involving hundreds of personnel. Similarly, clinical personnel who are not involved in the F2F visit are working remotely, including establishing and preparing for virtual visits, conducting patient outreach support, and managing care transitions for patients. More extensive work innovations in this area can be expected as the care delivery system shifts to a greater reliance on virtual care. Wearable devices and other remote patient monitoring tools support this growing trend to provide necessary services and care to patients beyond the traditional brick-and-mortar office setting.

Work Environment

Like any organization, ambulatory practices may experience challenges in the workplace. These issues are exacerbated by the often-frenzied work environment of an ambulatory practice. Ambulatory practices find value in developing protocols for a workplace that support an ideal working environment. While some practices may have a productive atmosphere naturally, being proactive in creating a positive working environment benefits everyone at the practice in the long term. Box 7.1 lists elements of an effective workplace policy, as espoused by the AMA. Consider the case study at the end of this chapter about managing disruptive physician behavior to further understand the topic of work environment.

Centralization

Ambulatory practices may operate in isolation; however, they are increasingly becoming connected to a larger healthcare entity. The integration may be a function of possession; the practice may be, for example, owned and operated by the local hospital. The nature of the ownership structure, however, is not a requirement for centralization for ambulatory practices. Technology creates the connective tissue that spans the healthcare delivery system, transcending matters of governance, management, and ownership. Figure 7.6 offers a lens into the multitude of touch points for the patients' journey.

BOX 7.1   ELEMENTS OF AN EFFECTIVE WORKPLACE POLICY

- Describe the management's commitment to providing a safe and healthy workplace.
- Show the staff that their leaders are concerned about bullying and unprofessional behavior and that they take it seriously.
- Clearly define workplace violence, harassment, and bullying, specifically including intimidation, threats, and other forms of aggressive behavior.
- Specify to whom the policy applies (i.e., medical staff, administration, patients, employees, contractors, vendors, etc.).
- Define both expected and prohibited behaviors.
- Outline steps for employees to take when they feel they are a victim of workplace bullying.
- Provide contact information and a clear process for confidentially documenting and reporting incidents.
- Prohibit retaliation and ensure privacy and confidentiality.
- Document training requirements.

SOURCE: American Medical Association. (2021). *Bullying in the health care workplace.* https://www
.ama-assn.org/system/files/2021-02/workplace-aggression-report.pdf

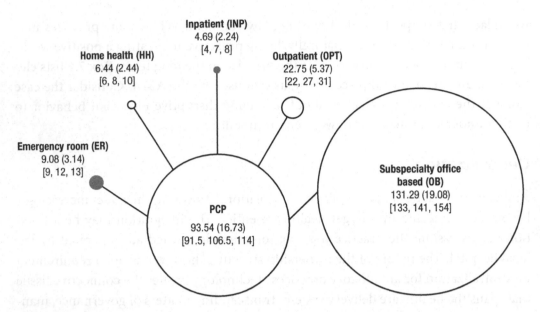

FIGURE 7.6 Weekly health care events for adult patient panel.

SOURCE: Rossi, M., & Balasubramanian, H. (2018). Panel size, office visits, and care coordination events: A new workload estimation methodology based on patient longitudinal event histories. *MDM Policy & Practice, 3*(4), 11. https://doi.org/10.1177/2381468318787188

NOTE: Mean (*SD*) of observed weekly event counts by event type for a panel of 2,000 patients (patient panel based on the Medical Expenditure Panel Survey] 2011 over 18 years of age and reporting a usual use of primary care). The second line gives the 50th, 75th, and 90th percentiles in brackets.
PCP, primary care provider

Ambulatory practices are considered vital to managing the care of patients; the structure and deployment of staff to support this mission is ever evolving. A system that consistently supports the care of patients requires a different framework than employing a staff member to work from 8:00 a.m. to 5:00 p.m. on weekdays; healthcare cannot be relegated to fit within a business day. A practice operating alone may fall victim to functioning with limited staff capacity whereby tasks are not reliably performed. Pooling of staff resources through centralization offers an alternative model. There is, however, proven value to cultivating relationships with patients, as familiarity with patients' needs can lead to better outcomes. For ambulatory practices, a balance must be struck between scale and intimacy. The perfect staffing model does not exist.

The demands of ambulatory practice management require a nimble, flexible structure for a support team. Avoiding fragmented care is a crucial consideration in constructing a staffing model for ambulatory care. To this end, staffing the ambulatory enterprise is evolving from personnel operating in isolation at disjointed sites to teams deployed effectively to work within systems of care leveraged to meet patients'

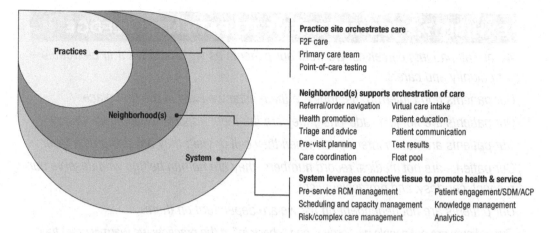

FIGURE 7.7 Sample staffing model for centralized support of ambulatory practices.

F2F, face-to-face; RCM, revenue cycle management; SDM, shared decision making; ACP, advanced care planning

needs. Figure 7.7 displays a sample staffing model designed to balance the value of the clinician–patient relationship with a system-level, coordinated, scalable strategy dedicated to holistic care for the community.

Service

This chapter is primarily devoted to the mechanics of staffing; however, the importance of personnel of an ambulatory practice in establishing, cultivating, and furthering a culture of service excellence cannot be overstated. The often-hectic environment of an ambulatory practice may lead to focusing on protocols and procedures to ensure efficiency and effectiveness, but it is vital to elevate service above all else. Hiring and retaining personnel who are committed to patient-centered care is crucial. Exhibit 7.2 offers a pledge that articulates the practice's commitment to patients. The pledge is a reminder of the most important service an ambulatory practice provides—hiring and managing a team of personnel who exemplify the commitment they have to caring deeply and fully for their patients.

CONCLUSION

In summary, the care team of an ambulatory practice consists of clinicians and support personnel dedicated to ensuring high-quality patient care and service. The clinical and business infrastructure required to manage in this environment necessitates a well-coordinated team of individuals who have been delegated specific roles, responsibilities, and accountabilities.

EXHIBIT 7.2 'COMMITMENT TO PATIENTS' PLEDGE

We are all patients ourselves. We treat our patients as we would want to be treated – with dignity and care.

Our patients don't interrupt us; they are the reason we exist in the first place.

Our patients are not just "add-ons"; they are the most important people in our day.

Our patients are not an interruption when they call or visit; they are doing us a favor.

Our patients are not medical record numbers; they are human beings who deserve our respect, courtesy, and professionalism.

Our patients are not dependent on us; we are dependent on them.

Our patients are not people we "arrive" and "check in" at the practice; we warmly greet them.

Our patients have a choice; we recognize and appreciate that they chose us.

Our patients aren't just more work to do; they honor us by allowing us to provide care to them.

DISCUSSION QUESTIONS

1. What are some reasons that new training might have to be conducted with ambulatory practice personnel?

2. What are some of the benefits and drawbacks of using a pooled staffing model instead of a practice operating alone?

3. Why, as the practice expands, do the functions performed by the administrative personnel become more specific?

4. Why do you think "meeting practices" is one of the three aspects of team performance in the Conceptual Model of Interprofessional Team Performance?

5. How might the COVID-19 pandemic change the job description of certain ambulatory practice personnel?

REFERENCES

American Medical Association. (2021, May 5). *Policy research perspective*. https://www.ama-assn.org/system/files/2021-05/2020-prp-physician-practice-arrangements.pdf

American Nursing Association. (n.d.). *Scope of practice*. https://www.nursingworld.org/practice-policy/scope-of-practice/

Berry, L., Selders, K., & Wilder, S. (2003). Innovations in access to care: A patient-centered approach. *Annals of Internal Medicine, 139*, 568–574. https://doi.org/10.7326/0003-4819-139-7-200310070-00009

Gottschalk, A., & Flocke, S. A. (2005). Time spent in face-to-face patient care and work outside the examination room. *Annals of Family Medicine, 2005*, 488–493. https://doi.org/10.1370/afm.404

Institute of Medicine. (2010). Institute of Medicine (US) Committee on the Robert Wood Johnson Foundation Initiative on the Future of Nursing, at the Institute of Medicine. (2011). *The future of nursing: Leading change, advancing health*. National Academies Press (US).

Warde, C. M., Giannitrapani, K. F., & Pearson, M. L. (2019). Teaching primary care teamwork: A conceptual model of primary care team performance. *The Clinical Teacher, 17*, 249–254. https://doi.org/10.1111/tct.13037

Case Study

Disruptive Behavior

Iris Grimm
  Physician & Leadership Coach
  Master Performance, Inc.
  Atlanta, Georgia

A Manager's Difficult Day

"After Dr. Wright left the room, I couldn't help but breathe a sigh of relief. It wasn't easy, but I got through the meeting and, maybe, got my point across to him about the negative impact his behavior was having on our staff."

Here's how things got to this point: Soon after I took this job as Practice Manager of Medical Associates, I was told by the practice partners that any personnel issues and staff communication that pertained to Dr. Wright would be handled through me. In other words, if a staff member has a problem with Dr. Wright, they will share it with me, and I will talk with him about it. And when Dr. Wright has an issue with a staff member, he will communicate it with me, and I will mediate it between him and the particular individual. I remember being taken aback by that statement because he was nothing but a gentleman in my interactions with him.

But then the first issue arose: A medical assistant refused to work with him on the afternoon that his regular associate was out, and I had to step in and calm emotions.

A couple of months later, while I was on vacation, Dr. Wright attempted to handle a complaint by the tech who confided to him that she was unhappy at the practice. Instead of deferring the conversation until my return, he said to her bluntly, "Well, if you are unhappy, you have to leave." Unfortunately, she took his response literally and submitted her resignation letter a week later. Within a couple of weeks, she took a similar position at a competing practice.

Unless I convince Dr. Wright to take positive steps to improve his dealings with staff, I worry that the practice partners will consider disciplinary action against him or even terminate his employment, even though he is consistently the group's highest producing physician each quarter.

I think I got my points across to him, and we were able to agree to some guidelines and goals to turn around his disruptive behavior and prevent future adverse incidents with staff.

Discussion Question: The Practice Manager is relieved that the meeting went well; how would you have handled the meeting?

Physician and leadership coach Iris Grimm shares key points to manage disruptive behavior:

Invite. Invite the physician to a conversation to address the recent "situation with a staff member." Avoid judgmental or accusatory terms, such as *incident, your behavior*, and so on. Instead, describe the topic in a neutral statement focused on a positive outcome. Ideally, the meeting should occur in a neutral setting, such as a conference room or someone else's office, where you don't get interrupted. If you meet at your office, avoid sitting behind your desk; instead, sit in a seating area or across each other without a physical barrier.

Disarm. At the onset of the meeting, attempt to reduce tension and forestall a defensive reaction by asking an open-ended, off-topic question such as, "How are things going in your practice?", "How was your weekend?" and the like, depending on how well you know the physician so far. Then, launch into the reason for the meeting, but do so in a nonconfrontational, neutral manner, such as saying, "It's been brought to my attention that a staff member complained about your management style. Since there are always two sides to a story, I'd like to begin by getting your version of the event(s), so we can figure out a way to prevent this from happening again."

Stay Neutral. Focus on asking open-ended questions about the what, when, and where of the incident. Avoid questions that start with "why." They can come across as defensive. Instead, replace why with the term "what was the reason . . ."

Observe. Don't just listen to the words, but also pay close attention to the nonverbal communication. Be present to the physician's tone of voice, body language, facial expression, and demeanor. They help you sense the energy behind the words. If the physician becomes irritated or defensive, point it out with compassion, repeat the meeting's intention, and if necessary, allow a short break to calm down emotions.

Take Notes and Repeat Key Responses. Ask the physician for permission to take notes during the conversion. Ideally, write down the notes during speaking pauses. Along with eye contact and positive body language, taking notes can help convey that you want to get their side of the matter. Repeat key comments and explanations to clarify that you understood them as intended.

Dig Deeper. If the physician makes broad statements like, "I told them a thousand times . . .", ask for a more precise description.

Disapprove the Behavior, Not the Person. Instead of commenting that the physician has been disruptive, focus on the behavior and its impact on others.

Summarize. At the meeting's conclusion, verbally summarize the physician's statements so that they feel heard.

Seek Agreement on Next Steps. Finally, seek the physician's buy-in to solutions. These may include brainstorming with you at a subsequent meeting, scheduling skills coaching sessions with you or an outside expert, and/or exploring outside resources, such as online classes or educational articles. The more you can keep the physician out of defensiveness, and the more you stay on a solution-focused conversation, the more cooperative and open-minded (s)he will be. In some cases, you might seek a three-way meeting with you, the physician, and the employee to work out solutions, but that is a judgment call you'll have to make depending on the personalities and issues involved.

Ultimately, the physician must be coachable and willing to improve. Be sure to monitor their progress, and don't hesitate to offer further suggestions and interventions if you see little or no progress being made. Most physicians value working in a smooth-running practice environment where the interpersonal conflicts that may occasionally occur (we are all human after all) are not ignored but rather addressed promptly and fairly. The winners will be you, your physicians, staff, and patients.

Bonus: When you start at a new practice, make a proactive effort to build strong relationships with all physicians. Get to know them, ask them what matters to them, build trust. And should you ever have to lead a crucial conversation such as that which is described in the case, it will make it smoother.

ACRONYMS

AAAHC: Accreditation Association for Ambulatory Health Care
ABN: Advance Beneficiary Notice
ACO: Accountable care organization
ACSC: Ambulatory Care Sensitive Condition
AHA: American Hospital Association
AHRQ: Agency for Healthcare Research and Quality
AKS: Anti-kickback statute
AMA: American Medical Association
AMC: Academic medical center
APC: Ambulatory payment classifications
ARRA: American Recovery and Reinvestment Act of 2009
ASC: Ambulatory surgery center
ASCQR: Ambulatory Surgical Center Quality Reporting
ATB: Aged trial balance
BCBS: Blue Cross Blue Shield
BLS: Bureau of Labor Statistics
BMI: Body mass index
CAHPS: Consumer Assessment of Healthcare Providers and Systems
CBC: Complete blood count
CDC: Centers for Disease Control and Prevention
CDI: Clinical Documentation Improvement
CF: Conversion factor
CHIP: Children's Health Insurance Program
CIN: Clinical integrated network
CMA: Certified medical assistant
CMS: Centers for Medicare and Medicaid Services
CMS-1450: Centers for Medicare and Medicaid Services 1450 Claim Form
COVID-19: Novel Coronavirus of 2019
CPT®: Current Procedural Terminology
CT: Computed tomography
DRG: Diagnosis-related group

DRO: Days in receivables outstanding

E&M: Evaluation and Management

ED: Emergency department

EDI: Electronic data interchange

EHR: Electronic health record

EKG: Electrocardiogram

F2F: Face-to-face

FC: Fixed costs

FDA: Food and Drug Association

FFS: Fee for service

FQHC: Federally qualified health center

FTE: Full-time equivalent

GDP: Gross domestic product

GPCI: Geographic practice cost index

HCC: Hierarchical Condition Categories

HCPCS: Healthcare Common Procedure Coding System

HIPAA: Health Insurance Portability and Accountability Act

HITECH: Health Information Technology for Economic and Clinical Health Act

HMO: Health maintenance organization

HPV: Human papillomavirus

ICD: International Statistical Classification of Diseases and Related Health Problems

ICD-10-CM: International Classification of Diseases, Tenth Revision, Clinical Modification

IOM: Institute of Medicine

IPA: Independent practice association

IT: Information technology

JCAH: Joint Commission on Accreditation of Hospitals

JCAHO: Joint Commission for the Accreditation of Healthcare Organizations

KPI: Key performance indicator

LLC: Limited liability company

LPN: Licensed practical nurse

LVN: Licensed vocational nurse

MA: Medical assistant

Medicare PFS: Medicare Physician Fee Schedule

MP: Malpractice

MSO: Management services organization

NAM: National Academy of Medicine

NAMCS: National Ambulatory Medical Care Survey

NCQA: National Committee for Quality Assurance

NCR: Net collection rate

NHAMCS: National Hospital Ambulatory Medical Care Survey
NPI: National Provider Identifier
NPSR: Net patient services revenue
NQF: National Quality Forum
OPD: Outpatient department
OPPS: Outpatient Prospective Payment System
OR: Operating room
P&L: Profit and loss
PC: Physician compensation
PC: Professional corporation
PCMH: Patient-centered centered medical home
PDCA: Plan, Do, Check, Act
PE: Practice expense
PEST: Political, Economic, Social, and Technological
PHO: Physician hospital organization
PM: Practice management
PMPM: Per member per month
POS: Place of service
PPACA: Patient Protection and Affordable Care Act
PPO: Preferred provider organization
PREM: Patient-reported experience measure
PRO: Patient-reported outcome
PROM: Patient-reported outcome measure
PSR: Patient service representative
QPP: Quality Payment Program
RASCI: Responsible, Accountable, Support, Consulted, and Informed
RBRVS: Resource-based relative value scale
RCM: Revenue cycle management
RCT: Randomized controlled trial
RE: Revenue per encounter
RHC: Rural health clinic
RN: Registered nurse
RVU: Relative value units
SBNA: Scheduled but not arrived
SDOH: Social determinants of health
SMART: Specific, Measurable, Attainable, Relevant, and Time-bound
SME: Subject matter expert
SOAP: Subjective, objective, assessment, and plan
STEEPLE: Social, Technology, Economic, Environmental, Political, Legal, and Ethical
SWOT: Strengths, weaknesses, opportunities, and threats

TJC: The Joint Commission
TOL: Top of license
TPS: Toyota Production System
VCE: Variable costs per encounter
WHO: World Health Organization
WRVU: Work relative value unit

GLOSSARY

Advanced Practice Provider: A licensed, nonphysician provider with a scope of practice defined at the state level in the United States. Also called "midlevel provider" and "physician extender," providers may include physician assistants or advanced practice registered nurses (e.g., nurse practitioners, certified nurse specialists, certified nurse-midwifes, certified registered nurse anesthetists).

Allowable: Expected reimbursement rates, or "allowable rates," for procedures and services as defined by the agreement between the ambulatory practice (or individual physician) and the insurance company for the amount that is allowed to be collected for the procedure or service.

Ambulatory Care Sensitive Conditions: Health conditions for which effective outpatient care can reduce or prevent the need for hospitalization or avoid complications or more severe presentations of a disease.

Appointment Duration: The length of a given appointment as defined by the time allocated on the appointment schedule; typically, durations are set for new and established patients, for example, 15 minutes for established patient and 30 minutes for new patients.

Benchmarks: Performance metrics that are expressed as measurable standards which may be used as a basis for comparison.

Care Team: All members involved in patient care, including clinicians, staff, and families.

Care Transitions: Coordination of care between providers or settings, such as a patient discharged from the hospital to be subsequently cared for in the ambulatory setting.

Clinical Intake: A formal process in an ambulatory practice that is consistent across specialties and includes collection of vital signs, asking questions, administering health screenings, and/or other clinical preparation needed for the encounter with the provider. Also referred to as "rooming."

Consolidation: When organizations merge or are acquired; in healthcare, this may be prompted by a desire for cost savings or improved care coordination.

Core Competency: A competitive advantage or defining strength that sets an organization apart from its competition.

Denial: When a healthcare claim is not approved for payment.

Donabedian Model: A conceptual framework for the assessment of quality of care through the lenses of structure, process, and outcome. Named for Dr. Avedis Donabedian, who was a physician and health services researcher.

Eligibility: Meeting all requirements for insurance coverage.

Emphasis on information technology interoperability: A focus on health information systems that work together to advance healthcare delivery.

Environmental Analysis: An assessment of an organization's internal capabilities and competencies as well as a reflection on the external landscape.

Escalation: An action taken to raise an alert about a patient's care. An ambulatory practice, for example, may have an escalation protocol for a patient who complains of chest pain during a phone call to schedule an appointment.

Financial Clearance: Collecting insurance information such as the insurance company or health plan and accompanying identification numbers and gathering appropriate details to determine the financially responsible party.

Fixed Costs: Expenses that remain stable regardless of the ambulatory practice's volume; these costs may include the practice's rent, malpractice, and information technology costs.

Gross Charge: The price for each unit of service of an ambulatory practice; the charge may get lowered to an allowable.

Huddle: Stand-up meetings performed once a day with a team to discuss the upcoming day and review the day prior; typically, no more than 10 minutes.

Institute of Medicine: An independent nonprofit organization that provides unbiased, authoritative advice to the public and decision-makers, also known as the National Academy of Medicine.

Journey Map: The process of visualizing and documenting a process from the patient's perspective; for example, the patient's steps from the moment the need for a clinical visit is identified.

Latent Conditions: An unidentified condition that underlies or adjoins a process; an unrecognized design flaw that may lead to an active failure in a healthcare setting.

Lean Production: A production methodology focused on eliminating waste.

Mergers and Acquisitions: Also known as M&A, where one organization is acquired by another or merges (joins together) with a similar organization.

Mobile Health: The provision of healthcare over mobile devices, such as smartphones, tablets, and computers.

Organizational Chart: A diagram that highlights various roles, responsibilities, and reporting relationships in an organization.

Outcomes: The events that occur as the result of an intervention.

Overhead: A measure of a practice's ability to use operating expenses to leverage its revenue-generating assets—clinicians; typically expressed as a percentage, the calculation is expenses divided by revenue.

Patient-centered: A dimension of healthcare quality that focuses on patient needs.

Patient-Reported Outcome Measures: Any report of the status of a patient's health condition that comes directly from the patient without interpretation of the patient's response by a clinician or anyone else, according to the National Quality Forum.

Patient Panel: A group of patients assigned to one specific physician or team, often measured as patients who have been seen at least once during a certain time period (e.g., previous two years). Used commonly in primary care.

Payer: An insurance company or other entity that pays for or arranges for the payment of a medical or healthcare service or procedure.

Population: A distinct group of individuals.

Portal: A secure, encrypted online communication platform that provides patients with 24/7 access to personal health information and other functions such as appointment scheduling and messaging.

Prior Authorization: A process through which physicians obtain advance approval from a patient's insurance company for a service or item; also known as a pre service authorization request.

Process Improvement: Using clinical data measurement for care delivery to identify best practices and incorporate them into workflows.

Profit: Revenue less expenses—also known as net income.

Provider-based Clinic: Services provided in hospital outpatient departments that are clinically integrated into the hospital.

Psychological Safety: The belief and understanding that one will not be punished for sharing ideas, questions, and concerns.

Referral: The recommendation of a medical professional to see another professional (e.g., a primary care "refers" a patient to a gastroenterologist to be assessed for recurring stomach pain) or receive certain services; alternatively, a referral may refer to an administrative requirement by an insurance company or health plan that must be fulfilled by the *referring* physician in order for the *receiving* physician to be paid.

Registration: Enrolling a patient's name and identifying information at the practice for treatment, operations, and payment.

Revenue Cycle: All administrative and clinical functions that contribute to the capture and management of patient service revenue.

Rise of consumerism: The increase in the acquisition and consumption of goods and services and corresponding expectations for better service, convenience, affordability, and transparency by consumers.

Scope of Practice: The services and procedures that a healthcare provider is permitted to undertake in keeping with their professional license; in the United States, it is regulated at the state level.

Self-Scheduling: The ability for patients to schedule healthcare appointments online.

Shift From Free for Service to Alternative, Value-Based Payment Models: The transition from a traditional healthcare model which assigns reimbursements based on the services provided to a newer, value-based model where reimbursement is contingent on quality of care provided.

Social Determinants of Health: According to the Centers for Disease Control and Prevention, the five key social determinants of health are healthcare access and quality, education access and quality, social and community context, economic stability, and neighborhood and built environment.

Stakeholders: The patients, physicians, employers, insurance companies, and others who have a vested interest in healthcare.

Standing Orders: Protocols prepared by medical professionals to carry out various medical services in advance of assessing the patient based on the patient's symptoms and/or complaints; for example, a patient who fell and cannot twist their ankle may have an X-ray taken prior to a more extensive examination by the physician.

Strategic Alternatives: Different courses of action that an organization can choose to pursue.

Strategic Intent: An organization's overarching purpose.

Strategic Plan: The alignment of a business's coordinated strategies into a cohesive document and plan.

Telemedicine: The practice of caring for patients in a remote setting with the use of technology.

Teleworker: Someone who practices or works from home.

Template: A guide or pattern that can be used as an example.

Top of License: The collective initiatives related to leveraging education and training at its fullest extent have emerged using the term *top of license*.

Triple Aim: The triple goal of improving experience of care, enhancing population health, and reducing per capita costs of healthcare, promulgated by the Institute of Healthcare Improvement's Donald Berwick, MD, Thomas Nolan, MD, and John Whittington, MD.

Wait List: A list of those persons waiting for an appointment.

INDEX

AAAHC. *See* Accreditation Association for Ambulatory Health Care
ABN. *See* Advance Beneficiary Notice
ACA. *See* Affordable Care Act
access
    to appointments, 18
    to healthcare, 17, 158, 217
    to insurance, 16, 22–23, 154
    to telemedicine, 150
account follow-up representatives, 211
accountability, 47, 103, 104–105, 121
accountable care organizations (ACOs), 21–22, 65, 73–74
accounts receivables, 179
Accreditation Association for Ambulatory Health Care (AAAHC), 81
ACOs. *See* accountable care organizations
ACSCs. *See* ambulatory care sensitive conditions
action plan, 46–47, 52
active failures, 79, 90, 91
activity-based cost monitoring, 187
administrative support personnel, 209–212
Advance Beneficiary Notice (ABN), 128
advanced practice providers, 27, 147, 200, 201, 208
Affordable Care Act (ACA), 22, 73–74
aged trial balance (ATB), 179, 180, 185
Agency for Healthcare Research and Quality (AHRQ), 17, 77, 102
AHA. *See* American Hospital Association

AHRQ. *See* Agency for Healthcare Research and Quality
AKS. *See* anti-kickback statute
allowables, 164, 166–167, 182
AMA. *See* American Medical Association
ambulatory care, 1
    ancillary care providers, 63
    centralization, 219–221
    "commitment to patients" pledge, 221, 222
    community health centers, 12, 14, 63
    convenience clinics, 63, 65
    cost of healthcare, 9–10
    daily employee workload ranges, 212
    definition of, 1–2
    delivery systems, 10–15
    elements for evaluation in, 43
    employment, 25–27
    engagement of U.S. government, 7–9
    freestanding emergency departments, 62
    growth of, 27–29
    health insurance, 5–7
    historical context of, 2, 4–10
    hospital outpatient departments, 12, 13, 14, 62, 175, 176
    hospital-based practice, 215
    impact of technology, 19–21
    improvement strategies, 99–105
    industry trends, 15–23
    large ambulatory practice, 215
    mid-size ambulatory practice, 214
    organizational structures, 21–22
    patient demand management, 114

ambulatory care (*cont.*)
  patient engagement, 16–17
  physician office and hospital outpatient
      visits, 2, 3–4, 203–204
  physician offices, 11–12, 63
  preventative care, 17–18
  public health departments, 13, 15
  scheduling management, key performance
      indicators in, 121, 122–124
  services offered by, 57–58
  small ambulatory practice, 213
  value-based care, 18–19, 20
Ambulatory Care Improvement Guide
      (CAHPS), 102
ambulatory care sensitive conditions
      (ACSCs), 83, 84–85
Ambulatory Health Care Accreditation
      program (TJC), 81, 92
ambulatory payment classifications
      (APCs), 177
ambulatory surgery centers (ASCs), 8, 62,
      66, 175, 176
Ambulatory Surgical Center Quality
      Reporting (ASCQR) Program, 102
American Association of Medical
      Clinics, 6
American College of Physicians, 81
American College of Surgeons, 79, 81
American Hospital Association (AHA), 22,
      81, 150
American Medical Association (AMA), 8,
      12, 81, 171, 219
American Medical Group Association
      (AMGA), 6
American Nursing Association, 207
American Recovery and Reinvestment Act
      of 2009 (ARRA), 20, 138
AMGA. *See* American Medical Group
      Association
ancillary care providers, 63
anti-kickback statute (AKS), 71–73, 192
APCs. *See* ambulatory payment
      classifications

appointment(s)
  access to, 18
  confirmation, 114, 121
  durations, 117
    benchmarks for, 118
  schedule/scheduling, 95–96,
      114–121
  template, 117, 119
  triage, 112
  types, 117
ARRA. *See* American Recovery and
      Reinvestment Act of 2009
arrival, patient, 126, 210
  check-in, 126–127
  clinical intake, 129–130
  common forms used during, 128
  rooming, 127–129
  telemedicine, 139–140
ASCQR. *See* Ambulatory Surgical Center
      Quality Reporting Program
ASCs. *See* ambulatory surgery
      centers
assignment of benefits form, 128
ATB. *See* aged trial balance
automated self-scheduling, 120
automated wait list, 120–121

balance sheet, 194
Balanced Budget Act of 1997, 139
balanced scorecard, 48
Barton, Clara, 79
behavior change, 53
billers, 211
billing requirement for in-office ancillary
      services exception, 69
billing service, 180
Blackwell, Elizabeth, 79
board of directors, 59, 60
board of trustees, 35
bonus payments, 165
brainstorming, 49, 52, 225
breakeven analysis, 188–189
budget, 195–196

CAHPS. *See* Consumer Assessment of Healthcare Providers and Systems
CAHPS Clinician and Group CAHPS (CG-CAHPS), 94
CAHPS Home Health Care (HHCAHPS), 94
CAHPS Outpatient and Ambulatory Surgery Survey (OAS CAHPS), 94
Canadian Medical Association, 81
capabilities, organizational, 40–41, 45
capacity building, 35
care coordination, 134–135
care management team tasks, virtual *vs.* face-to-face, 209
care team, 217
  associates, 211
  conceptual model of primary care team performance, 218
care transitions, 135
CDC. *See* Centers for Disease Control and Prevention
CDI. *See* clinical documentation improvement
Centers for Disease Control and Prevention (CDC), 2, 18, 202
Centers for Medicare and Medicaid Services (CMS), 12, 21–22, 24, 62, 85, 88, 94, 102, 128, 177
  adoption of CPT, 171
  criteria for reasonable and necessary item/service, 125
  Primary Care First program, 158
centralization, 219–221
certified medical assistants (CMAs), 208
certified nurse specialists, 207
CG-CAHPS. *See* CAHPS Clinician and Group CAHPS
change leadership, 53
charitable clinics, 6
check-in, 126–127
Children's Health Insurance Program (CHIP), 22

CHIP. *See* Children's Health Insurance Program
CINs. *See* clinically integrated networks
circle of trust, 100
claim follow-up, 179–180
claim submission, 177, 179
clinical documentation improvement (CDI), 170
clinical intake, 129–130, 139–140
clinical integration, 22
clinical laboratory personnel, 208
clinical support personnel, 208–209
clinically integrated networks (CINs), 22
clinicians, 51, 53, 114, 130, 131, 200–202
  billing under Medicare PFS, 201
  compensation plans for, 189–190
    cost treatment, 191–192
    revenue treatment, 190–191
  role in inter-encounter work, 137
  staffing
    and community needs, 202–204
    external benchmarks, 205–207
    internal benchmarks, 204–205
    regulatory environment, 207
    reimbursement, 207
CMAs. *See* certified medical assistants
CME. *See* continuing medical education
CMS. *See* Centers for Medicare and Medicaid Services
Cochrane, Archie, 79
coder, 177
Codman, Ernest, 78–79
coinsurance, 168
collaboration, 52, 54, 218
commercial accountable care organizations, 74
communication, 46, 48, 52, 101, 137, 218
  appointment confirmation, 121
  care coordination, 134
  care transitions, 135

communication (*cont.*)
  in exam rooms, 100
  inter-encounter, 135–136
  personnel, 210
  plan, 47
  platform, 113, 148, 158
  and referrals, 126
community
  -based ambulatory care, 8
  leaders, participation in strategic
      planning, 36
  needs, and clinician staffing, 202–204
community health centers, 12, 14, 63, 202
community hospitals, outpatient utilization
      in, 13
compacts, 126
compensation, 39, 67, 68, 185, 216
  plans, for clinicians, 189–190
    cost treatment, 191–192
    revenue treatment, 190–191
  relationship, 66
competencies, organizational, 41
confidentiality, 97, 100
consultation centers, 2, 4
Consumer Assessment of Healthcare
      Providers and Systems (CAHPS), 102
consumer demand, and telemedicine,
      149–150
consumerism, 92–94
continuing medical education (CME), 216
convenience clinics, 63, 65
coordinated care, 6
copayment, 168
core competencies, 41
corporate practice of medicine
  and integrated care, 73
  and ownership, 58
  prohibition, 63–65
corporations, 59–60
  friendly professional corporations, 64
  general business corporations, 60, 64
  nonprofit corporations, 60–61
  professional corporations, 60, 64

cost(s)
  activity-based cost monitoring, 187
  budgeted, 195
  and clinician compensation plans,
      191–192
  cost-volume-profit visualization, 193, 194
  fixed costs, 185–187
  personnel costs, 186
  step-fixed costs, 186–187
  variable costs, 187
COVID-19 pandemic, 15, 139, 154, 218
  change in volume of visits to U.S.
      ambulatory practices after, 152
  and mental health, 159
  and telemedicine, 150, 152, 153
CPT. *See* Current Procedural Terminology
      codes
credentialing, 134, 207
Current Procedural Terminology (CPT)
      codes, 164, 167, 171–172, 182
customer intimacy, 159
customer service representatives, 211

daily template, 116
dashboards, 48, 181
data
  electronic data interchange, 179, 181
  patient data verification, 112
  for performance improvement, 102
  referral, 205
days in receivables outstanding (DRO),
      180, 185
deductible, 168
delivery systems, ambulatory care, 10–15
Deming, W. Edward, 79, 103, 140, 141
demographic information, 111, 112
denied claims, 182, 183–184
design thinking, 95, 96
designated health services, 65–66, 68–69
diagnosis coding, 172–173
diagnosis-related groups (DRGs), 9
direct primary care, 158
dispensaries, 2, 4, 5, 6

disruptive behavior, 223–225
doctors' offices, 175
documentation
    of clinical encounter, 132
    of messages, 135
    service documentation, 170–171
Donabedian, Avedis, 79, 80, 81, 92, 93
Donabedian model, 80, 81–82, 89
double booking, 115
DRGs. *See* diagnosis-related groups
DRO. *See* days in receivables outstanding

early adopters, 53
ED. *See* emergency department
Eddy, David, 79
edit report, 177
education, staff, 216–217
EHR Incentive Program, 20, 151
EHRs. *See* electronic health records
electronic consults, 126
electronic health records (EHRs), 19–20,
        21, 127, 130, 131, 135, 136, 137, 138,
        151, 170
eligibility process, 112, 169
emergency department (ED)
    ambulatory care sensitive visits, 85
    freestanding emergency departments, 62
emotional intelligence, 54–55
empathy, 55, 129
employee workload, daily, 212
employment in ambulatory sector, 25–27
encounter, 130–132, 210
    documentation of, 132
    huddles, 130, 131
    SOAP (subjective, objective, assessment,
        and plan) framework, 131
environmental analysis, 39–40
    external analysis, 42–44
    internal analysis, 40–42
episode of care, 164
equipment leases, 68
error report, 177
escalation protocols, 112–113, 137

eVisit, 157
exam rooms, 133
    design, 98, 99, 100–101
    escorting patients to, 127–129
expenses, 185
    and budget, 195–196
    fixed costs, 185–186
    profit, 187–194
    step-fixed costs, 186–187
    variable costs, 187
external analysis, 42–44

facilities and maintenance staff, 211
faculty practice plan, 176
False Claims Act, 66
Families First Coronavirus Response
        Act, 150
family presence in exam rooms, 100
FDA. *See* Food and Drug Administration
Federally Qualified Health Centers
        (FQHCs), 9, 63, 175
feedback, 48, 51, 52
fee-for-service (FFS) payment system, 10,
        73–74, 164
Feinstein, Alvan, 79
FFS. *See* fee-for-service payment system
finance and accounting staff, 210
financial analysis, 42
financial and administrative policies
        form, 128
financial clearance, 111, 169
financial management, 163
    expenses, 185–187
    financial statements, 194–196
    patient financial responsibility, 168
    revenue, 163–169
    revenue cycle, 169–185
financing/funding, 6–8
fishbone diagram, 143
Five Forces (Porter), 161
Five S, 142–143
fixed costs, 185–187
flat monthly payment, 164

Flexner Report (1910), 6
focus groups, 44, 51
Food and Drug Administration (FDA), 83, 149
FQHCs. *See* Federally Qualified Health Centers
freestanding emergency departments, 62
friendly professional corporations, 64
front office staff, 211
Futures Wheel, 48–49, 50

gap analysis, 41, 44
general business corporations, 60, 64
general partnerships, 58–59
global fee/payment, 164
goals, strategic, 46
governing body, 34–35, 46, 47, 51
    capacity building, 35
    stakeholder identification and engagement, 36
    surveillance, 35
GPO. *See* group purchasing organization
gross charges, 166, 167–169
group cohesion, 53
group practices, 6, 7, 10, 11, 62, 200
    in-office ancillary services exception, 68–71
    investment, and anti-kickback statute, 72
group purchasing organization (GPO), 148

HCAHPS. *See* Hospital Consumer Assessment of Healthcare Providers and Systems
HCPCS. *See* Healthcare Common Procedure Coding System
healthcare costs, 9–10, 23–25
healthcare spending
    as a share of gross domestic product, 24–25
    in United States (2019), 26
health centers, 12, 14, 63, 202
health departments, 5, 6, 7, 9, 13, 15
Health Information Technology for Economic and Clinical Health (HITECH) Act, 20

health insurance, 5–7, 8, 113, 165
    access to, 22–23
    for ambulatory-only procedures, 10
    coinsurance, 168
    coverage, and income-to-poverty ratio, 24
    denied claims, 182, 183–184
    employer premiums, deductibles, and wages, 16
    features of health plans by firm size, 151
    information, 111, 112
    insurance referral, 121, 124, 125
    managed care, 10
    number of uninsured people and uninsured rate among nonelderly population, 23
    and telemedicine, 150, 151, 154
    third-party payments, 7, 8
Health Insurance Portability and Accountability Act (HIPAA) of 1996, 128, 171
health maintenance organizations (HMOs), 8, 74
Health Professional Shortage Area (HPSA), 154
Health Resources and Services Administration, 63
Healthcare Common Procedure Coding System (HCPCS), 171
HHCAHPS. *See* CAHPS Home Health Care
Hill-Burton program, 6
HIPAA. *See* Health Insurance Portability and Accountability Act of 1996
HITECH. *See* Health Information Technology for Economic and Clinical Health Act
HMOs. *See* health maintenance organizations
home location, 175
Hospital Consumer Assessment of Healthcare Providers and Systems (HCAHPS), 93–94
Hospital Services and Construction Act of 1946, 6

hospital(s), 158
  -based ambulatory practice, 215
  -employed physicians, 11–12
  Joint Commission on Accreditation of
      Hospitals (JCAH), 81
  leadership in, 51
  Medicare spending on hospital outpatient
      services, 12, 14
  Minimum Standard for Hospitals, 79
  off-campus outpatient hospital, 175
  on-campus outpatient hospital, 175
  outpatient departments/clinics, 4, 5, 7, 8,
      12, 13, 14, 62, 175, 176
  outpatient utilization in community
      hospitals, 13
  outpatient visits, 2, 3–4, 203–204
  rental of space, 67–68
HPSA. See Health Professional Shortage
    Area
huddles, 130, 131
human capital, 39
human factors of medical errors, 91
human resources, 199
  administrative support personnel,
      209–212
  care team, 217, 218
  centralization, 219–221
  clinical support personnel, 208–209
  clinicians, 200–208
  compensation, 216
  daily employee workload ranges, 212
  disruptive behavior (case study),
      223–225
  education and training, 216–217
  job description, 214, 216
  labor pool, 199
  management, 212–213
  performance management, 216
  service, 221
  staff, 210–211
  staffing patterns, 200–201
  teleworkers, 218
  top-of-license, 217
  work environment, 218–219

ICD. See International Statistical
    Classification of Diseases and
    Related Health Problems
ICD-10-CM. See International Classification
    of Diseases, Tenth Revision, Clinical
    Modification
incident-to billing, 27, 28
income statement, 194–195
income-to-poverty ratio, and health
    insurance coverage, 24
independent practice associations (IPAs), 21
indigent clinics, 5
information technology (IT) staff, 210
in-office ancillary services exception,
    68–71, 72
Institute of Medicine (IOM), 9, 17, 78, 87,
    91, 217
insurance. See health insurance
insurance follow-up representatives, 211
insurance referrals, 121, 124, 125
integrity, and process improvement,
    103, 105
inter-encounter, 134
  care coordination, 134–135
  care transitions, 135
  communication, 135–136
  test results, 136–137
internal analysis, 40–42
International Classification of Diseases,
    Tenth Revision, Clinical
    Modification (ICD-10-CM),
    172–173
International Statistical Classification
    of Diseases and Related Health
    Problems (ICD), 172
IOM. See Institute of Medicine
IPAs. See independent practice
    associations
Ishikawa diagram, 143
IT. See information technology staff

JCAH. See Joint Commission on
    Accreditation of Hospitals
job description, 214, 216

Joint Commission, The (TJC), 81–82, 91, 102, 110, 136
Joint Commission on Accreditation of Hospitals (JCAH), 81
joint ventures, 61
journey mapping, 96, 98
Juran, Joseph, 79
just culture, 102

Kaizen, 143
Kanban, 143
Karnofsky Performance Index, 83

latent conditions, 79, 90–91
leadership, 33, 49, 51, 99, 101, 102, 103. See also strategy
    dyad, 51, 52
    emotional intelligence, 54–55
    and management, 53
    and patient experience, 98–99
    roles and responsibilities, 51–52
    strategic planning skills, 52–53
lean production, 140, 142–143
lean thinking, 82, 142
legal requirements of organizations, 58, 63
    corporate practice of medicine prohibition, 63–65
    self-referral prohibitions, 65–71
Lemonaid Health, 146–149, 159–161
    business model, 148
    competitors, 154, 155–157
    and consumer demand, 151
    mission of, 147
    partnerships, 149
    patient flow at, 147
liability insurance, 153
licensed practical nurses (LPNs), 208
licensed vocational nurses (LVNs), 208
licensing, 58, 153
limited liability companies (LLCs), 61
limited partnerships, 59
LLCs. See limited liability companies
local government officials, working with, 44–45

location requirement for in-office ancillary services exception, 69
LPNs. See licensed practical nurses
LVNs. See licensed vocational nurses

mail order prescriptions businesses, 152
malpractice, 136, 207
managed care, 9–10
management, 53, 212–213
management services agreement, 64–65
management services organizations (MSOs), 64–65
manager-managed limited liability companies, 61
market trends, identification, and evaluation of, 44
MAs. See medical assistants
master template, 116
Mayo, Charles, 6
Mayo, William, 6
Medicaid, 7, 8, 22
medical assistants (MAs), 208
medical errors, 87, 89–91
Medical Group Management Association, 2, 6
medical homes, 17, 74, 134
Medical Payment Advisory Commission (MedPAC), 12, 25, 27
medical practice management, 6
medical records release form, 128
medical training programs, 8
Medicare, 7, 8, 58, 71, 87, 167, 173
    accountable care organizations, 21–22, 65, 73–74
    beneficiaries, mix of clinicians in encounters of, 27
    Physician Fee Schedule, 176, 201
    resource-based relative value scale, 9, 173–174
    spending on hospital outpatient services, 12, 14
    and Stark Law, 65, 66
    for telemedicine services, 139
    wellness visits, 49

medications, 90, 152, 153–154, 187, 207

MedPAC. *See* Medical Payment Advisory Commission

member-managed limited liability companies, 61

mental health
and insurance coverage, 154
primary care practice preparedness to manage patients with mental illnesses, 160
in telemedicine, 146, 158–159

mentor relationships, 216

mergers, 45, 46

messages, 135

metrics, 141–142

Minimum Standard for Hospitals, 79

mini-registration, 111

mission, organizational, 33, 35, 37, 39

mobile units, 175, 202

monitoring systems, 104–105

MSOs. *See* management services organizations

multispecialty group practices, 10

NAM. *See* National Academy of Medicine

NAMCS. *See* National Ambulatory Medical Care Survey

National Academy of Medicine (NAM), 17

National Ambulatory Medical Care Survey (NAMCS), 8–9, 202

National Association of Clinic Managers, 6

National Association of Community Health Centers, 12

National Committee for Quality Assurance (NCQA), 102, 132, 134

National Health Service Corps Program, 8

National Healthcare Quality and Disparities Report, 102

National Hospital Ambulatory Medical Care Survey (NHAMCS), 8–9, 202

National Patient Safety Goals, 91, 92

National Quality Forum (NQF), 102

NCQA. *See* National Committee for Quality Assurance

NCR. *See* net collection rate

neighborhood health clinics, 7, 8

net collection rate (NCR), 184

net patient services revenue (NPSR), 165

NHAMCS. *See* National Hospital Ambulatory Medical Care Survey

99213 CPT code, 172

non-covered services, 168

nonprofit corporations, 60–61

Notice of Privacy Practices, 128

NPSR. *See* net patient services revenue

NQF. *See* National Quality Forum

OAS CAHPS. *See* CAHPS Outpatient and Ambulatory Surgery Survey

objectives, strategic, 46

OEO. *See* Office of Economic Opportunity

off-campus outpatient hospital, 175

Office of Economic Opportunity (OEO), 7–8

on-campus outpatient hospital, 175

online pharmacies, 153, 154

OPDs. *See* outpatient departments

operational excellence, 159

operational flexibility in exam rooms, 101

operations, ambulatory practice, 109
arrival, 126–130
electronic health records, 138
encounter, 130–132
inter-encounter, 134–137
Lemonaid Health (case study), 146–161
performance improvement, 140–143
post-encounter, 133–134
pre-encounter, 110–126
stages of, 110
standard operating procedures and metrics, 141–142
technology, 137–140
telemedicine, 138–140

OPPS. *See* Outpatient Prospective Payment System

order sets, 113

organizational capabilities, 40–41, 45

organizational competencies, 41

organizational structure, 21–22, 57–58,
        200, 212
    ambulatory settings and services, 61–63
    hospital-based practice, 215
    integrated care, 73–74
    large ambulatory practice, 215
    legal organization, 58
        corporations, 59–61
        limited liability companies, 61
        partnerships, 58–59
    legal requirements, 58, 63
        anti-kickback statutes, 71–73
        corporate practice of medicine
            prohibition, 63–65
        self-referral prohibitions, 65–71
    mid-size ambulatory practice, 214
    ownership, 58
    services offered by practice, 57–58
    small ambulatory practice, 213
outcomes, and healthcare quality, 78, 79, 80,
        81, 82, 83–84, 89, 93
out-of-network, 168
out-of-pocket maximum, 168
out-of-pocket payments, 127, 148, 168–169
outpatient departments (OPDs), 4, 5, 6, 7, 8,
        12, 13, 14, 62, 175, 176
Outpatient Prospective Payment System
        (OPPS), 12, 176, 177, 178
overbooking of appointment slots, 115
overhead, 185, 187, 192–194
ownership, 58, 66, 176, 219

P&L. *See* profit and loss statement
partnership(s), 58
    agreement, 59
    with external providers, 45
    general partnerships, 58–59
    limited partnerships, 59
patient care services, 69–70
patient demand, 114, 115, 121, 202, 205
patient engagement, 16–17
patient experience, 77–78, 92, 129. *See also*
        quality, healthcare
    consumerism, 92–94

    design, 94–99
    expectations, 94
    improvement strategies, 99–105
    moments of truth, 93
    and physical environment, 97
patient financial responsibility, 168
patient flow, 147, 210
patient history form, 128
patient identification, 110–111
patient identifier, 110
patient outreach, 113
patient panel
    benchmarks, 205–206
    weekly healthcare events for, 220
patient portals, 113
patient service representatives (PSRs),
        126, 211
patient-centered care, 17, 221, 222
patient-centered medical homes (PCMHs),
        17, 74, 134
patient-centeredness, 95
patient-encounters test, 70
patient-reported experience measures
        (PREMs), 83–84
patient-reported outcome measures
        (PROMs), 83–84
payer mix, 166–167, 174
PCMHs. *See* patient-centered medical
        homes
PDSA. *See* Plan-Do-Study-Act cycle
per member per month (PMPM) fee, 10
"per member per month" payment, 164
performance improvement, 104, 140–143
performance management, 216
personal services arrangement
    and anti-kickback statute, 72–73
    exception, 66–67
personnel costs, 186
PEST (Political, Economic, Social, and
        Technology) analysis, 42, 43, 49
PFS. *See* Physician Fee Schedule
PHOs. *See* physician-hospital organizations
physical environment, 97
Physician Fee Schedule (PFS), 176, 201

physician groups, 11, 62
physician-hospital organizations (PHOs), 21
physicians, 185, 200
    collaboration of leaders with, 52
    disruptive behavior, 223–225
    hospital-employed, 11–12
    office-based, adoption of EHRs by, 21
    participation in strategic planning, 36
    physician offices, 11–12, 62
        outpatient visits, 2, 3–4, 203–204
    physician-administrator dyads, 212
place of service (POS) codes, 174–176
Plan-Do-Study-Act (PDSA) cycle, 79,
        103, 143
PM. *See* practice management systems
PMPM. *See* per member per month fee
poka yoke, 143
polyclinics, 5
population health management strategy,
        35, 41
portfolio analysis, 42
POS. *See* place of service codes
post-encounter, 133–134, 140
PPOs. *See* preferred provider organizations
practice management (PM) systems, 21,
        138, 184
pre-encounter, 110
    appointment confirmation, 121
    appointment schedule, 114–121
    referrals, 121, 124–126
    registration and scheduling, 110–114
    telemedicine, 139
preferred provider organizations (PPOs),
        74, 167
PREMs. *See* patient-reported experience
        measures
preventative care, 17–18, 49
pre-visit, 169
Primary Care First program, 158
prior authorizations, 125
privacy, 100, 153
procedure coding, 171–172
process, and healthcare quality, 80, 81, 89, 93
process improvement tools, 103

product leadership, 159
professional associations, 44, 81, 205, 209
professional corporations, 60, 64
profit, 185, 187, 194–195
    breakeven analysis, 188–189
    clinician compensation plans, 189–190
        cost treatment, 191–192
        revenue treatment, 190–191
    cost-volume-profit visualization, 193, 194
    overhead, 192–194
profit and loss (P&L) statement, 194–195
PROMs. *See* patient-reported outcome
        measures
prospective payment system, 9, 12, 176,
        177, 178
provider matching, 119
provider supply, 114, 150–152
provider-based clinics, 176
PSRs. *See* patient service representatives
psychological safety, 51
public health, 4–5, 6. *See also* COVID-19
        pandemic
public health departments, 13, 15
public health services, 15

QPP. *See* Quality Payment Program
quality, healthcare, 19, 77, 78–81, 92.
            See also patient experience; safety
    domains, 78
    Donabedian model, 80, 81–82, 89
    improvement, 88–89
        strategies, 99–105
    lean thinking, 82, 142
    measures, 82–85, 88–89
    pioneers of, 79
    reporting, 85–87, 89
quality of life, 83
Quality Payment Program (QPP), 85–87
Quality Trilogy, 79
Quest Diagnostics, 149

radiology technicians, 208
RASCI (Responsible, Accountable, Support,
        Consulted, and Informed) tool, 48

RBRVS. *See* resource-based relative value scale

RCM. *See* revenue cycle management

Reason, James, 79, 90, 91, 102

receptionists, 126, 211

referral(s), 44, 121, 124–126, 211
  for clinical care, 121, 124
  data, and clinician capacity, 205
  insurance referrals, 121, 124, 125
  referral coordinators, 126
  Stark prohibition on, 68–69

registered nurses (RNs), 208

registration, 110–114, 210

regulations
  and clinician staffing, 207
  telemedicine-related, 153–154

reimbursement, 7, 9
  and clinician staffing, 207
  denied claims, 182, 183–184
  management, 182–185
  models, 164–165
  rates, 167
  for telemedicine, 153, 154

relative value unit (RVU), 173

remote care, 209

rental of space, 67–68

reporting, quality, 85–87, 89

resource-based relative value scale (RBRVS), 9, 173–174

revenue, 163–164
  and budget, 195–196
  and clinician compensation plans, 190–191
  gross charges, 167–169
  net patient services revenue, 165
  payer mix, 166–167
  reimbursement models, 164–165

revenue cycle, 169, 170
  claim follow-up, 179–180
  claim submission, 177, 179
  diagnosis coding, 172–173
  personnel, 210
  place of service designation, 174–176

pre-visit, 169
procedure coding, 171–172
reimbursement management, 182–185
resource-based relative value scale, 173–174
service documentation, 170–171

revenue cycle management (RCM), 169, 180–181

revenue optimization staff, 211

RHCs. *See* rural health clinics

risk payments, 164–165

RNs. *See* registered nurses

rooming, 127–129

rural health clinics (RHCs), 8, 9

RVU. *See* relative value unit

safety, 77–78, 87, 89–92. *See also* quality, healthcare
  exam room, 100
  improvement strategies, 99–105
  National Patient Safety Goals, 91, 92
  and patient identification, 111
  pioneers of, 79
  Systems Engineering Initiative for Patient Safety (SEIPS) 2.0 model, 90

satellite departments, 62

SBAR (Situation-Background-Assessment-Recommendation) technique, 103

SBNA. *See* scheduled-but-not-arrived rate

scenario analysis, 42

scheduled-but-not-arrived (SBNA) rate, 189

scheduling, 110–114, 210
  appointment, 95–96, 114–121
  automated self-scheduling, 120
  blocks, holds, and freezes, 116–117
  inquiries, questions for, 120
  management, key performance indicators in, 121, 122–124
  provider matching, 119
  strategic booking, 115
  team, 211
  wait lists, 120–121

scheduling horizon, 115

scheduling template, 116, 140

scope of practice, 199, 207, 208

scribes, 132

SDOH. *See* social determinants of health

SEIPS. *See* Systems Engineering Initiative for Patient Safety 2.0 model

self-awareness, 54

self-check-in, 126, 127

self-referral laws, 71, 192. *See also* anti-kickback statute (AKS)

self-referral prohibitions, 65–66
   in-office ancillary services exception, 68–71
     personal services exception, 66–67
     rental of space, 67–68

self-regulation, 54

self-scheduling, 120

self-service registration, 111, 112

service documentation, 170–171

service excellence, culture of, 221

session template, 116

shareholders, 59

Shattuck, Lemuel, 4–5

Shewhart, Walter, 79

SMART (Specific, Measurable, Attainable, Relevant, and Time-bound) principles for goal setting, 46

SMEs. *See* subject matter experts

SOAP (subjective, objective, assessment, and plan) framework, 131

social determinants of health (SDOH), 18, 19, 112

Social Security Amendments of 1965, 7

sole proprietorships, 58

solo practices, 200

SOPs. *See* standard operating procedures

space, rental of, 67–68

specialists, 5, 6, 10, 124, 125, 126, 202

specialty societies, 205, 209

split billing, 176

sports medicine, 44–45

staff per FTE physician ratio, 209

stakeholder analysis, 42

stakeholders, 33, 39, 48, 96
   identification and engagement of, 36
   input of, 44
   and quality improvement, 89
   role and responsibilities of, 52–53

standard operating procedures (SOPs), 141–142

standing orders, 130

Stark Law, 65–66, 67, 68, 69–71, 73

statement of cash flows, 195

statement of financial position. *See* balance sheet

STEEPLE (Social, Technology, Economic, Environmental, Political, Legal, and Ethical) criteria, 49

step-fixed costs, 186–187

storytelling, 101

strategic alternatives, 44–46, 49, 51, 52, 53

strategic booking, 115

strategic foresight, 48–49

strategic intent, 37, 38, 39, 40, 49, 51, 160

strategic plan, 33, 35, 37–39, 49, 51
   action plan
     establishing, 46–47, 52
     execution of, 47
   development, 39–48
   draft, distribution of, 51–52
   environmental analysis, 39–44
   evaluation elements in ambulatory care setting, 43
   evaluation of progress, 48
   pillars, 38, 39
   strategic alternatives, 44–46, 49, 51, 52, 53
   strategic goals and objectives, 46
   strategic planning skills of leaders, 52–53
   third-party consultants for, 34, 36

strategy, 33, 37. *See also* leadership
   ambulatory practice leaders, 36
   capacity building, 35
   governing body, 34–36
   stakeholder identification and engagement, 36
   surveillance, 35

strategy-to-performance gap, 47
structure
    and healthcare quality, 80, 81, 89, 93
    and patient experience, 96–97
subject matter experts (SMEs), 103
substantially-all test, 69–70
super groups, 11
supervision requirement for in-office
        ancillary services exception,
        68–69
surveillance, 35
sustainability of performance improvement
        initiatives, 103–105
SWOT (Strengths, Weaknesses,
        Opportunities, and Threats)
        analysis, 42
systems engineering, 140
Systems Engineering Initiative for Patient
        Safety (SEIPS) 2.0 model, 90

takebacks, 164–165
team(s)
    -based approach, for performance
        improvement, 102–103
    building, 52–53
    care management team tasks, 209
    care team, 217
    scheduling team, 211
TeamSTEPPS (Team Strategies and Tools to
        Enhance Performance and Patient
        Safety), 103, 104
technical factors of medical errors, 91
technology, 113, 219. *See also* telemedicine
    for check-in, 126, 127
    impact on ambulatory care, 19–21
    and quality measurement, 83
    and quality reporting, 87
    and registration process, 112
    role in operations, 137–140
    use in encounter, 130
    use in scheduling, 115, 117, 119, 121
telemedicine, 64, 138–140, 202
    barriers to, 153

competitive landscape, 154–158
consumer demand, 149–150
and health insurance, 150, 151, 154
Lemonaid Health, 146–161
market, 149–152
mental health in, 158–159
provider supply, 150–152
regulatory and reimbursement
        environment, 153–154
teleworkers, 218
test results, 130, 136–137
third-party consultants for strategic
        planning, 34, 36
third-party payments, 7, 8
TJC. *See* Joint Commission, The
TOL. *See* top-of-license
top-of-license (TOL), 217
Toyota Production System (TPS), 82,
        140, 142
TPS. *See* Toyota Production System
training, staff, 216–217
triage, 112
Triple Aim, 93

United States Public Health Service, 6
urgent care clinics, 62, 64, 175
user-centered design, 97

value stream mapping, 143
value-based care, 18–19, 20
value-based payment programs, 85
value-chain analysis, 42
values, organizational, 33, 35, 37, 39
variable costs, 187
virtual primary care, 158
vision
    organizational, 33, 35, 37, 39
    strategic, for performance improvement,
        101–102

wait lists, 120–121
waiver form, 128
walk-in clinics, 94, 175

wearable devices, 218
wellness visits, 49
Wennberg, John, 79
WHO. *See* World Health Organization
work environment, 218–219

work relative value units (WRVU), 190, 191, 205
workplace policy, 219
World Health Organization (WHO), 84, 172
WRVU. *See* work relative value units

Printed in the United States
by Baker & Taylor Publisher Services

Printed in the United States
by Baker & Taylor Publisher Services